The Psychology of Dental Patient Care — a common-sense approach

The Psychology of Dental Patient Care — a common-sense approach

By

Dr Ruth Freeman

Senior Lecturer in Dental Public Health, School of Clinical Dentistry, The Queen's University of Belfast

2000

Published by the British Dental Association
64 Wimpole Street, London, W1M 8AL

ISBN 0 904588 55 6

Printed and bound by
Dennis Barber Ltd, Lowestoft, Suffolk

Preface

Those aspects of patient management that matter most to patients have not been covered well or at sufficient depth in the dental literature. This book, characterised by the 'common-sense approach', aims to remedy that.

The central theme of the book is that 'dental health care is a two-person endeavour', not something that one person does to another. It offers practical strategies and a framework of theory to underpin them. This approach is informed by the author's own experience in practice and her expertise in behavioural science.

Frequent vignettes, many with the charming immediacy of verbatim transcription, illustrate the workings and effects of various psychological principles. These are balanced by clear expositions of those theories. Some technical terms are used, and explained, because to access information in another discipline it is necessary to be able to understand its concepts and use its vocabulary.

The book deals with barriers, or 'resistances' to dental care, and shows that there are some which originate with the healthcare professional. In this, as in other aspects of the dentist–patient relationship, an equality is proposed. Thus a patient's anxiety may be mirrored by a dentist's stress; concerns about fee levels may be mutual; time pressures may operate on both individuals. Considerable attention is paid to the reality of undue stress on dental professionals and the possibility of reducing this by the approaches suggested.

The author offers systems for conducting effective interviews, for differentiating between phobic and merely anxious patients and for recognising avoidance behaviours. She outlines the CLASS framework (Context, Listening, Acknowledgement, Strategy, Summary) widely used in medicine for effective communication. She reminds readers of the classic 'Tell–Show–Do' method.

The book also points out that whilst dentists think of dental symptoms in physical terms, patients experience those symptoms in their own psychological and social context. Understanding this allows more effective help to be given. An adolescent who begins to resist the 'health directed' behaviour of brushing to maintain gum health, may respond to the 'health related' benefit of fresh breath. This is an example of a 'common-sense' approach, but illustrates and conceptualises why and how it works. Readers of the book will become able to see other applications of the principles described that can apply to their own daily practice.

The author looks at the three-person treatment alliance that must be forged when a child is the patient. The phenomenon of regression is described in which anxiety will produce behaviour characteristic of a younger age group. Awareness of this makes it easier for the professional to make an appropriate response. The effect of the parent's own fears and beliefs about dentistry and oral health must be taken into account. This is debated in the chapter entitled 'The Case for Mother in the Surgery'.

Chapter 2 contrasts professional and lay attitudes. Patients vary widely in translating the presence of oral symptoms into action to access care. Professional and lay attitudes are often widest apart in defining the need for treatment. Understanding this mismatch is essential if the unmet oral health needs of those who only attend in an emergency are to be provided.

It has been widely found that simply giving health advice produces disappointing results. Although clear about the constraints that time and fee levels may impose upon professionals, the case is made for using the motivational interviewing technique. This is used with the 'Stages of Change' model which identifies stages of contemplation or readiness to act. While making it clear that some means of providing information is essential, this section looks at how patients can form an effective and equality-based alliance for change with their dental professionals.

Throughout the book the author shows awareness of the danger of 'burnout' in overstressed dentists. The lasting benefit of this book may be treatment alliances with patients who have become responsible for their own dental health through more rewarding and less fraught experiences for both parties.

Elinor Parker
Associate Editor, *BDJ*

Contents

Introduction — The common-sense* approach

This introduction is entitled 'The common-sense approach'. There are those who may be critical of this title. 'Common-sense', they will say, 'devalues the psychological understanding of dentistry'. They will have none of it. They will discard the ideas and concepts presented here as being anecdotal and unscientific. Furthermore, they will say that scientific research and evidence-based criteria show that common-sense is worthless. However to think of common-sense as something which should be discarded and of little value, is to ignore the importance of knowledge which has already been acquired. This knowledge has always been known by those within a particular group, and as such has a value of its own. Hence, another school of thought exists in which the notion of common-sense knowledge is highly valued.

Common-sense versus evidence

How can this tussle between research findings and evidence-based criteria on the one hand and common-sense (acquired knowledge) on the other be resolved? Could it be that common-sense based on acquired knowledge and research findings are really two sides of the same coin? Support for this suggestion may be sought by considering two pieces of research. The first of these examined why adolescents intended to take sugar in hot drinks.[1] It showed that the adolescents did so because the beverages tasted nicer. The second research project investigated heart rate and dental anxiety.[2] It showed that anxious patients' heart rates were higher during treatment compared with patients who were not fearful of dentistry. Both of these research results

---

*Common-sense: practical intelligence, sagacity. English Dictionary. London: Penguin Books 1997.

could be described as common-sense — since from personal experience putting sugar in hot drinks does make them taste nicer and from personal knowledge and education, it is known that increased heart rate is a physiological expression of anxiety.

Common-sense (acquired knowledge) should perhaps be thought of differently. Maybe it should be thought of as a special type of knowledge which is based upon an individual's life experiences. By thinking in this way, acquired knowledge may reflect research findings as well as permitting the marrying of common-sense with psychological ideas of patient management.

The aim of this book is to re-acquaint dental health professionals with their acquired knowledge, as well as providing information about patient management, leading, it is hoped, to a comprehensive understanding of the psychology of dental patient care. In order to achieve this aim the chapters are connected to one another with two main themes pervading the book. The central theme is the notion that dental health care is a two-person endeavour. This must be based upon an equality between participants[3] which represents the second and subsidiary theme. It is necessary, therefore, to consider each aspect of patient care from both patient and dental health professional perspectives. Thinking in this way allows the development of patient care to be based upon an equality of status between participants.

In order to achieve this patient management goal, dental health professionals must have an understanding of what happens within the dentist–patient relationship. They must know about the determinants of dental health attitudes and behaviours and how these affect dental attendance. In addition, they must feel proficient in their communication and motivational skills so that they may be able to use this information to assist patients to access, accept and comply with dental health care and preventive health advice. The chapters address these issues in patient management. This is not to say that the chapters represent a 'how-to-do-it series' but it is hoped that dental health professionals may be able to make some use of the suggestions or ideas so that their patient management goals may be accomplished.

The chapters

The first three chapters look at various models of the dentist–patient interaction. This is necessary since aspects of the dental health professional–patient interaction may lead to difficulties inherent in patients accepting dental health care. The first chapter examines the dynamic quality of the dentist–patient relationship. While several models have been suggested to explain the dentist–patient relationship the psychodynamic model proposed here postulates that dental health care is a two-person endeavour — the dentist and the patient. It acknowledges that to enable patients to accept dental health care in its widest sense, the dentist must admit to the potential inequalities within the interaction making adjustments as the needs arise. In this way the dentist within the interaction paves the patient's way to accept the dental treatment which is being offered and provided. The issue of inequality within the dentist–patient relationship is re-worked in Chapter 2.

Inequality in perception

The second model of the dentist–patient interaction is based upon the lay person's and dental professional's concepts of dental health. It becomes apparent that dental health professionals change during training (professionalisation) and this may mean that their concepts of dental health gradually change and become quite different from those of their patients. With professionalisation comes inequality in dental health care perception. For instance patients may access dental health care for reasons which may seem apparently divorced from their dental health status. An awareness of these differences between lay and professional perspectives of dental health allows the dentist to make adjustments within the dentist–patient relationship which may assist patients to access and accept dental healthcare.

If difficulties arise between dentists and their adult patients, then insurmountable problems may seem to exist with the treatment of children and adolescents. This subsidiary theme is first mooted in Chapter 3 and taken up again later in the book. When treating children the dental health professional interacts not only with the child but with the child's carer. It is the parent's wish for the child to have treatment which is uppermost and it is with the carer that the dentist must also make the treatment alliance. The issue of whether the parent remains in the surgery is thus important and is debated in the chapter entitled 'The Case for Mother in the Surgery'.

Wider perspectives

Chapters 1 to 3 examine the intricacies of the dentist–patient relationship, Chapters 4 and 5 look at the same issues from a wider perspective — the influences of psycho-social factors upon dental healthcare. Entering the second part of the book the reader is invited to explore psycho-social factors as determinants of dental health attitudes and behaviours. If patients are to be able to access and accept dental healthcare then it is necessary to understand the origins of health attitudes and behaviours. I will argue that those very psycho-social factors (such as demography, familial and peer group influences, dental anxiety status), which were instrumental in determining health routines and behaviours are those which form the greatest barriers to accessing dental healthcare (Chapter 5). The need to understand what is meant by the concept 'barrier' will be discussed. Two definitions of barrier are given: the first is a psycho-social definition and the second a dynamic explanation based upon the idea of 'resistance'. In Chapters 6 and 7, barriers to dental healthcare will be considered from both patient and dental health professional positions. Linking back into the central theme of dental care being a two-person endeavour and status equality, barriers to accessing care are, therefore, considered from a two-person perspective — that of the patient and that of the dental health professional. Appreciating that dental health professionals may unwittingly play a role in the construction of barriers, will allow the dentist to make adjustments to maintain an equality which will enable the patients to access and accept the care they offer and provide. In order to assist patients in this regard, the dentist must provide care which acknowledges and accommodates patients' worries, fears or concerns about the treatment itself or its outcome.

Effective communication

Armed with the awareness of what goes on within the dentist–patient relationship, the determinants of dental health attitudes and behaviours and their role with regard to assisting (enabling) or hindering (inhibiting) their patients accessing and accepting dental healthcare, the dental health professional is in a position to provide care which maximises equality between participants. However, at this juncture the dentist needs to have some practical skills. If the health professional is to find out what the patient feels about his or her dental health concerns, about treatment outcome and difficulties in complying with preventive dental regimes, then the dental health professional must be proficient and skilled in communication.

In Chapter 8, the effective communication strategy entitled 'CLASS'[4] is introduced to the reader as a technique useful in information retrieval. The acronym 'CLASS'[4] stands for the need for an empathetic Context for the interview, to Listen actively to the patient, to Acknowledge the patient's and one's own feelings about the interaction, to develop a preventive and restorative treatment Strategy and to provide a Summary of treatment and preventive options for the patient. I will suggest that by using the 'CLASS'[4] strategy dental health professionals will become more proficient in their communication skills. All the information needed to care, understand and negotiate preventive and treatment plans with patients will be obtained effectively.

Motivation

In Chapter 9, the central themes of dental healthcare being a two-person endeavour and the maintenance of equality with the professional–patient interaction are re-visited, but this time, with regard to helping patients to comply with preventive dental health advice. Chapter 9 brings together the earlier work to show how these may be incorporated into a system by which dental health professionals can motivate their patients to comply with preventive health care advice.

The reader is introduced to two strategies which may be used in this regard. The first strategy entitled 'motivational interviewing'[5] explores the issue of resistances or barriers to change. Re-working the concept of resistance, in this way allows the dental health professional to perceive the relevance of effective communication skills in his or her daily contact with patients. Using effective communication in conjunction with motivational interviewing, the practitioner is able to assess the patient's readiness to change. In other words, does the patient wish to change her dental health behaviours or is she in two minds (ambivalent) about it. By making this assessment with regard to the patient's readiness to change, the patient's wish to change can be slotted into a tailor-made programme based upon the 'Stages of Change Model'.[6] This model is divided into six different stages of behaviour change. The stages reflect the patient's readiness to change, the degree of ambivalence, the resolution of conflict, as well as the establishment and maintenance of the health behaviours. The stages reflect and hence provide a means of assessing progress from unawareness (precontemplation) through motivation (contemplation, preparation) to compliance (action, maintenance).

Motivating patients to change their health behaviours is a complex issue which relies upon the understanding and patience of health professionals. By using motivational interviewing together with the Stages of Change Model, dental health professionals can facilitate behaviour change in their patients. They do this by maintaining an equality between themselves and their patients. This equality allows patients to take charge of their own dental health decisions thereby enabling them to maintain their oral health status.

By increasing the awareness of dental health professionals to recognise the potential for inequalities within the dentist–patient interaction it is possible for dentists and members of the dental team to appreciate the complexities of the dentist–patient interaction. It is important that dentists understand the role of barriers with regard to the distortion of the equality of the dentist–patient relationship.

It has been suggested that barriers to compliance act to distort the relationship between the dentist and patient, reducing the patients' ability to align themselves with the dentist and accept the treatment offered (the treatment alliance). In this clinical scenario inequalities exist between patient and dentist. The dental health professional who is furnished with this acquired knowledge will have the ability to promote equality within the dentist–patient interaction thereby empowering and enabling the patients to comply with dental health advice so maintaining their own oral health status.

References

1 Freeman R, Sheiham A. Understanding decision making processes for sugar consumption in adolescence: factors affecting 'sound food choices'. *Community Dent Oral Epidemiol* 1997; 25: 228-232.
2 Freeman R. Using continuous heart rate monitoring to investigate anxiety and its communication within the dentist–patient interaction. *Psychol Health.* 1989; 3: 307-318.

3   Greenson R R. *The technique and practice of psycho-analysis.* London: Hogarth Press, 1989.
4   Buckman R, Korsch B, Baile W. *A practical guide to communication skills in clinical practice.* New York: Medical Audio Visual Communications Inc, 1998.
5   Rollnick S, Kinnersley P, Stott N. Methods of helping patients with behaviour change. *Br Med J* 1993; **307**: 188-190.
6   Prochaska J O, DiClemente C C. Stages and processes of self change of smoking: toward an intergrative model of change. *J Consul Clin Psychol* 1983; 5: 390-395.

A psychodynamic understanding of the dentist–patient interaction

The aim of continuous dental care is for dentists to be able to make contact with patients in an easy, accessible and acceptable manner. For patients who may be described as 'regular attenders' dentists have been able to form and maintain a 'treatment' relationship. This enables patients to accept the care which has been negotiated and offered.

For other patients it is impossible for the dentist or the dental team to contact them in either a physical or psychological way. Research suggests that these people remain non-compliant because they are too anxious, too impoverished and/or seem to be too disinterested to attend[1-3]. For whatever reason they are unable to use the dental care offered and provided by the dental team.

There are many ways in which dentists provide dental care for their patients and these techniques come under the umbrella of patient management. Methods of patient management are said to assist dentists in their work with patients by reducing stress not only in themselves but also in those individuals who form their dental teams. However despite increased awareness as to the importance of management skills, dental health professionals still experience stress, especially with patients who appear more demanding, anxious and who are sometimes described as 'difficult'. Patient management skills seem to have little bearing on the effect these patients can have upon the dental team. In fact dentists may state that even the mention of certain patients' names can lead to despondency. It would seem that some interactions with patients can stir up profound feelings. However unlike patients who have the potential to ventilate their anxieties and concerns, the dentist must keep his in check by reacting professionally within the confines of the dentist–patient relationship. In order for patient management to be successful it is important that dentists have an understanding of the ways in which patient interactions may progress.

Various models[4] have been suggested to explain the dentist–patient interaction. Some have suggested that a power differential[4–5] exists while others have formulated an explanation based upon psychodynamic ideas.[6–8] It has been suggested that using a psychodynamic model can help the clinician to appreciate that dental care is not one person working on another, but a two person endeavour involving adults working together toward a common health goal. The psychodynamic model assumes that when the dentist and patient are unable to work together toward the common health goal, difficulties may occur. It is proposed that an appreciation of the dynamics of the dentist–patient relationship will help to reduce occupational stress while enabling the patient to accept dental healthcare. The aim of this paper is to examine the dentist–patient relationship using a psychodynamic framework and to show its relevance for dentists and their patients in dental practice.

The psychodynamic explanation of the dentist–patient relationship[9]

From a psychodynamic viewpoint dental healthcare is a two-person endeavour. It is the dentist working with the patient and the patient being able to accept (use) the work (treatment) offered and provided by the dentist. It acknowledges that there is a uniqueness in the interaction for both dentist and patient while accepting the potential for inequalities within the interaction. Nevertheless it requires the health professional to remain flexible, to be able, as the need arises, to make adjustments in treatment plans thereby maximising status equality while minimising the potential for disruptions within the relationship. Benefits exist for the dental health professional when the equality between themselves and their patients is maintained. These include improved time and behavioural management skills, increased awareness of their patients' concerns and anxieties, the ability to readjust treatment plans and to provide patient-centred care.

There are three aspects of the psychodynamic model which must be considered in this regard. These are first the real relationship, secondly, the treatment alliance and thirdly, the transference.[9]

The real relationship

The real relationship is an equal and unique relationship between two adults. This is a genuine and realistic interaction in which the uniqueness of the dentist is complemented by the uniqueness of the patient. The interaction between them therefore has a distinction which belongs only to that specific patient who interacts with that particular dentist. Within the adult-to-adult equality of the relationship the dentist will have been chosen by the patient because of his clinical attributes and skills. The real relationship, in this regard, will remain unaffected by any anxieties or concerns the patient may have about dental treatment. Mrs W's interaction with her new dentist is a good example of the real relationship (Case 1). She experienced high dental anxiety and wished to find a dentist with good clinical as well as patient management skills. Her wish for a competent dentist was unaffected by her dental anxiety.

Case 1

Mrs W, a 25-year-old woman, had recently moved to a new town and was looking for a new dentist. She had been very pleased with her previous dentist with whom she had been able to manage her considerable dental anxiety. She would have continued to see him but for her new location. It was just too far to travel. She had asked about a dentist at her place of work and had been told that the dentist nearby had a good reputation. Mrs W decided to make an appointment. This was based upon the dentist's clinical reputation and patient management skills.

The treatment alliance

The treatment alliance is an equal relationship between two adults. However, while it possesses the same status equality of the real relationship, it differs. The treatment alliance is not only a development of the real relationship but is affected by the patient's anxieties and concerns with regard to accepting dental treatment. For the first time in the dentist–patient relationship the patient's concerns and anxiety about dental treatment seem to merge with the dentist's clinical and patient management skills. It is suggested that barriers to compliance, such as dental phobia, costs and so forth, act within the treatment alliance to distort the relationship between the dentist and patient. The intensity of anxiety, for instance, may render it impossible for the patient to depend upon, or align himself with, the dentist. The patient is unable to accept or use the treatment offered by the dentist.

The example of Laura (Case 2)shows how the intensity of the patient's anxiety can make the achievement of a treatment alliance difficult for both patient and dentist. Laura's anxiety was so intense that she was unable to depend upon the dentist (align herself with him) or use the dental care he was providing for her. However Laura's anxiety also affected the dentist. He too became unable to function within the treatment alliance, describing her as 'difficult'. Only after a realisation as to the inappropriateness of his reaction to the patient was he able to make adjustments and re-formulate his treatment plans in accordance with Laura's psychological and dental needs.

Case 2

Laura, a 25-year-old woman attended for dental treatment. She was anxious and delayed the start of treatment by using every means available to her. Despite being implored by the dentist and the nurse she finally refused to have any treatment at all, becoming distressed and tearful. After Laura left, the dentist complained 'difficult patients!'. However on reflection he acknowledged how uncomfortable he felt in response to the intensity of Laura's anxiety. When she came for the next visit he talked to her about her fears and concerns and Laura admitted that her anxiety had led to her being unable to sleep for nights. The dentist discussed with her why she was so anxious and subsequently by working together a treatment alliance was formed and together they were able to formulate a treatment plan.

The transference

The transference is quite distinct in its relationship characteristics but nevertheless inextricably linked to other aspects of the psychodynamic model. Like the treatment alliance the transference develops with time but unlike the real relationship or the treatment alliance this is not an interaction between adults. The transference represents the past. It is a repetition of previous emotionally important relationships which are inappropriately imposed by the patient upon the dentist. Therefore, as the transference represents the past, it sometimes becomes intrinsically associated with regression. Regression simply describes the psychological state of the patients as they change from being in an emotionally controlled to a less well controlled emotional state. Regression is associated with a change in relationship status. The interaction is no longer one of equality between adults but one between the dentist as 'parent' and patient as 'child' (Figure 1.1). Within the transference the adult patient will re-experience childhood memories and fears, which since they have become distorted with time are experienced as occurring in the present. The dentist may, therefore, be perceived as a caring parent whereas for other patients the dentist may be a powerful adult with the ability to cause fear or to harm.

The transference is particularly important in the management of dentally anxious patients since for them previous dental experiences are relived as if they were occurring in the here and now. The example of Mr B is illustrative (Case 3).

In this case, Mr B regressed from an emotionally controlled state outside the dental surgery to a less well controlled emotional state inside the

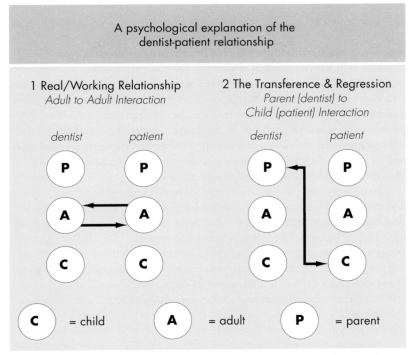

Figure 1.1 A psychological explanation of the dentist–patient relationship

dental surgery. The dentist's awareness of Mr B's feelings about dental treatment helped Mr B ventilate his concerns and anxieties. This was achieved because of the treatment alliance which existed, outside the transference. Mr B was able to use the information exchange with the dentist, together with the care offered by the dentist, as a result of the treatment

Case 3

Mr B was 55 years old. He was successful in his professional life and was considered to be assertive and impartial in his dealings with colleagues. Mr B was a regular dental attender despite being very frightened by the thought of dental treatment. While he remained assertive in his dealings outside the dental surgery, inside he admitted to such anxiety that he felt helpless like the little boy he once was. He openly talked of how he relived a childhood dental experience expecting each filling to be as painful as in the past.

alliance. The dentist had restored the adult-to-adult equality status in the dentist–patient relationship.

Applying the psychodynamic model to general practice

In order to illustrate the application of the psychodynamic model to general practice three basic models (Table 1.1) of the clinician–patient interaction proposed by Szasz and Hollender[6] will be explored. These models will be described separately. When they are brought together they provide an overall psychodynamic explanation of the dentist–patient interaction at different stages of the treatment encounter. Three general practice encounters will be used to illustrate how the dynamics of the dentist–patient relationship change with and within 'treatment' sessions.

The dental check-up visit: an example of the guidance–cooperation model

In the guidance–cooperation formulation of the dental check-up visit, Szasz and Hollender[6] described the relationship between the dentist and the patient not as one between two adults but one in which the dentist is the caring parent and the patient the cared-for child. While the guidance–cooperation model may explain the transference dimension of the check-up visit it ignores the treatment alliance and the real relationship. The attendance of

Three basic models of the dentist–patient interaction				
Model	Dentist's role	Patient's role	Clinical application	Prototype of model
Activity–passivity	does something to the patient	receives the treatment	operative dental treatment	parent to child
Guidance–cooperation	tells the patient what to do	obeys accordingly	dental check-up appointment	parent to child
Mutual–participation	advises and negotiates with patient	patient in equal partner care	negotiation treatment or preventive plans	adult to adult

Table 1.1 Three basic model of the dentist–patient interaction

the patient reflects the real relationship and treatment alliance. The patient re-attends because of the care afforded to her by the dentist. This is a reflection of the real relationship between dentist and patient. Since the patient has been able to use the dentist's care by attending, it also illustrates that the treatment alliance is operative. This reflects the adult-to-adult aspect of the guidance–cooperation formulation. Coleman and Burton have stated that when a patient attends for their check-up visit 'the patient knows something; dentist knows something'.[10]

In Case 4 Mrs R attended for her routine appointment. She thought as the dentist thought that there would be nothing to do. She also knew that something had to be done with her eye. Mrs R's response to her dentist's concern may be explained using the guidance–cooperation formulation. While acknowledging that she overcame a great anxiety she was, nevertheless, able to act on the dentist's guidance by cooperating and attending the eye department. She was able to do so because of the treatment alliance and her ability to use the information and care provided by the dentist.

Case 4

Mrs R attended for her usual check-up visit. She had assumed that nothing was wrong and was pleased when the dentist suggested that they should meet again in 12 months' time. However, the dentist noticed that a cyst at the corner of Mrs R's eye had become much larger since they had last met and mentioned his concerns. Mrs R got very angry. Nevertheless she phoned the surgery about four weeks later to thank the dentist. She had acted upon his advice and attended the eye department as an emergency. They had removed the lesion which was subsequently shown to be a lachrymal cyst. Mrs R had been very worried about it and was now reassured. She thanked the dentist for his interest in her general health.

The treatment session: an example of the activity–passivity model

The observation that during operative dental treatment the patient is passive and the dentist is active may be explained by the activity–passivity model: the patient must be passive and the dentist active so that dental treatment is possible. While the activity–passivity interaction is an example of the transference and regression it also contains aspects of the treatment alliance. If the treatment alliance were not in operation the patient would be unable to accept dental care as in the case of Laura. In Case 5 a woman patient attended for continuous dental care. Although having been a dental therapist, she felt it was as if she knew nothing of the dental procedure and the dentist knew everything.[10] Despite her disappointment in the dentist's patient management skills she remained a practice patient because of the real relationship and the treatment alliance.

This vignette shows how the treatment session interaction between dentist and patient is never static. Although Ms Z felt like a 'phantom head' (passive) when the dentist was preparing (active) the crown she nevertheless valued the dentist's clinical skills (the real relationship), the dentist's ability to care for her (transference) and, as she was able to use the treatment offered, remained a patient of the dentist (treatment alliance).

Case 5

Ms Z was having a crown prepared on an upper premolar. The dentist, who was known to her, gave the local anaesthetic and said little. After inquiring if the tooth was numb, the dentist started to work. Ms Z had not expected the dentist to explain the procedure but had been surprised by a sarcastic comment when she found the temporary crown high to bite on. She felt she was like a 'phantom head' just lying there. Ms Z acknowledged that patients 'don't go to her [*this dentist*] for her tact and diplomacy but for her considerable clinical skills'.

Negotiating preventive health goals: an example of the mutual-participation model

In the mutual-participation formulation two adults are working together for common dental health goals. This describes the negotiation of dental health goals suggesting that preventive dental care must be a two-person endeavour between adults.

The dentist, by recognising the potential for transference and the patient's wish to be cared for, acts to reinforce the treatment alliance within this mutual-participation formulation. This is achieved by encouraging the patient to be active and to use the information exchange to help her to participate as well as enabling her to take responsibility for her own dental health. In order to help the patient in this regard the dental health professional must be both active (providing information, advice) and passive (listening), making adjustments in order to maintain the treatment alliance. Techniques such as motivational interviewing and the stages of change model (see Chapter 9) may be used by the dental health professional to negotiate health goals. These techniques rely on the dentist and patient mutually participating in a joint venture to promote dental health.

Conclusions

Dental healthcare which acknowledges the role of the real relationship, the treatment alliance and the transference within a dynamic framework, will maintain the equality of the dentist–patient relationship. It is by an appreciation of the complexities of the dentist–patient interaction that the dental health professional will be able to enable patients not only to accept dental care but also to empower them to take responsibility for their own oral health.

References

1 Nuttall N. Review of attendance behaviour *Dental Update* 1997; **24**: 111-113.
2 Adams T, Freeman R, Gelbier S, Gibson B. Accessing primary dental care in three London boroughs. *Community Dental Health* 1997; **14**: 108-112.
3 Finch H, Keegan J, Ward K, Sen B B. *Barriers to the receipt of dental care. A qualitative study*. London: Social and Community Planning Research, 1988.
4 Sondell K, Soderfeldt B. Dentist-patient communication: a review of relevant models. *Acta Odontol Scand* 1997; **55**: 116-126.
5 ter Horst G, de Wit C A. Review of behavioural research in dentistry 1987-1992: dental anxiety, dentist-patient relationship, compliance and dental attendance. *Int Dent J* 1993; **43**: 265-278.
6 Szasz T S, Hollender M H. A contribution to the philosophy of medicine. *Arch Int Med* 1956; **97**: 582-592.
7 Freeman R. Communication, body language and dental anxiety. *Dent Update* 1992; **19**: 307-309
8 Burke F T J, Freeman R. Psychological aspects of patient management in dental practice. *Dent Update* 1994; **21**: 148-151.
9 Greenson R.R. *The technique and practice of psycho-analysis*. London: Hogarth Press, 1989.
10 Coleman H, Burton J. Aspects of control on the dentist-patient relationship. *Int Soc Lang* 1985; **51**: 75-104.

2

Reflections on professional–lay perspectives of the dentist–patient interaction

It is generally accepted that dentists know more about dentistry than their patients and that the dental treatment they provide is rooted in scientific and professional knowledge. To suggest otherwise would seem bizarre. Although treatment decisions are founded upon clinical and objective criteria, there is evidence to suggest that doing so at the expense of listening to patients' feelings may lead to difficulties in diagnosis, patient management and subsequent non-compliance with treatment plans.[1]

There is a tendency for dentists to discount their patients' worries while concentrating on professional and clinical matters. This concentration on clinical matters starts when the dental undergraduate changes from being a lay participant to being an active health professional. The process of professionalisation[2] requires the student to discard previously held lay views and accept professional ideas concerning health and causation of disease. As professionalisation continues the student's lay perspectives and health attitudes will be replaced by those of the profession. Professionalisation in this context maps out the process by which the student becomes a dentist. Once graduated the newly qualified dentist will have gained scientific knowledge, power, and autonomy characteristic of any professional group.[3]

This however only represents one side of the dentist–patient equation. The student's future general practice patients will not have experienced equivalent shifts in their dental health knowledge or related attitudes. The patient who enters the dental surgery may have a lay understanding of dental health matters similar to those held by the dentist prior to training. Within this professional–lay interaction the scene is set for a status differential to exist, characteristic of which, according to Coleman and Burton,[4] is that the dentist will know 'everything' (professional knowledge) and the patient will know 'nothing' (lay understanding).

To think of the dentist–patient interaction as one way traffic, with information and treatment flowing from dentist to patient, would be to ignore the dynamic quality of the relationship. By acknowledging that a dynamic interplay (see Chapter 1) exists provides the dental health professional with the opportunity for effective communication, information exchange and the negotiation of preventive and treatment goals.[1] Nevertheless the difficulties that can occur within the treatment alliance may cause disturbances in communication and information exchange with patients. This results from status inequalities within the dentist–patient relationship. The development of the status differential is associated with the professional and lay aspects of the dentist–patient interaction and is exacerbated by the tendency for the patient to perceive the practitioner as an adult figure and to feel like the child (s)he was once (see Chapter 1). Factors that may contribute to the development of this status differential also include how the participants view the impact of dental symptoms, how they feel symptoms are translated into accessing dental care as well as lay and professional perceptions of treatment need. These factors may have the potential to affect compliance because the same situation may be interpreted differently by dentists and their patients.

The aim of this chapter is to discuss each of the above factors in order to examine their potential to cause disruption in the treatment alliance. Understanding that dentists and patients perceive the same dental healthcare situation from different contextual frameworks (professional knowledge versus lay understanding) enables dentists to provide effective care instead of disappointing treatment outcomes and unachievable health goals.

Professional–lay perspective 1: impact of oral symptoms

What can be learned from Case 1? There seemed to be two different agendas with regard to Mrs P's symptoms — professional and lay. For the dentist the physical source of the pain and discomfort were of prime importance: for Mrs P her difficulty in eating, her reduced social contact with family and friends and her low spirits seemed to carry equal weight with the discomfort she experienced. It would be fair to say that Mrs P's quality of life had been affected by her oral symptoms. For Mrs P it was not only the physical impact of her oral symptoms but their psycho-social impact which particularly affected her.

The idea that physical symptoms can affect psychological functioning and social interaction is not new. It is almost to be expected in patients with atypical facial pain or burning mouth syndrome.[5–6] It has been suggested recently that equivalent feelings are experienced by patients with dental caries, periodontal disease and denture problems.[7–10]

Many of these dental patients have difficulties in interacting with family and friends. Some admit to feeling embarrassed when talking, eating or kissing and some will even avoid social occasions altogether. Such avoidance

Case 1

Mrs P was an 81-year-old widow. She complained of discomfort under her upper complete denture on eating. She had had these symptoms for several months but had attended now because eating was becoming 'impossible'. In fact she had cancelled a family outing as a result of her oral discomfort. She admitted the denture problem was getting her down.

The dentist examined Mrs P's mouth and found nothing clinically wrong. Symptomatic treatment was provided by way of easing of the denture. This afforded Mrs P some relief but she soon returned complaining of the same discomfort as before. The dentist was concerned about the physical origins of Mrs P's pain and referred her to the local dental hospital. Radiographic examination revealed the source of the pain and discomfort — two erupting canines.

behaviours will exacerbate feelings of anxiety and low-spiritedness resulting in even lower self-esteem and self-confidence.[11]

Patients, therefore, do not just perceive their oral symptoms in physical terms but also with regard to their quality of life. In this way lay perspectives of the impact of oral symptoms can be thought of as being analogous to a triangle of health,[12] being composed of physical, psychological and social dimensions (Figure 2.1).

Some value may be gained from thinking in this way as it provides a means of understanding why professional and lay perceptions of the impact of oral symptoms differ. The example of patient satisfaction with dentures is

Figure 2.1 The triangle of health

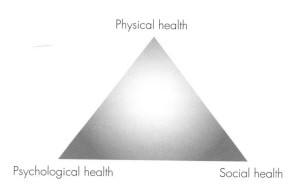

Physical health

Psychological health   Social health

illustrative in this regard. A recent study of patient denture satisfaction has shown that whilst patients' concerns were related to comfort (physical), aesthetics (psychological) and communication (social) factors, their dentists rated denture satisfaction in terms of the physical attributes of the denture.[10]

It would seem that rather than thinking in psycho-social terms dentists tend to restrict their focus to the physical impact dental symptoms have on their patients. For the dental health professional the impact of dental symptoms is perceived mainly in physical terms. This is important in the analysis of patient care, but for the patient symptoms have psychological, social as well as physical impacts.

Professional–lay perspective 2:
Translating oral symptoms into dental care
The diversity that exists between the perception of oral symptoms by professionals on the one hand and their impact on patients on the other, may provide an indication as to why some people attend routinely and others appear to attend only in an emergency. The issue of how the psycho-social impact of dental symptoms are translated into accessing treatment has been emphasised by Tickle *et al.*[9] They suggest it is the reporting of the physical symptoms together with the psycho-social factors that impact to provide the stimulus to access dental care.

How can such ideas relate to a group of patients for whom regular dental care has become part of a health routine and as such contributes to their quality of life? These patients routinely attend, but are not necessarily compelled to do so, because of the impact of physical symptoms. It has been proposed that these patients translate their dental care needs into regular attendance based upon their previous psycho-social experience of being cared for.[13] According to Coleman and Burton[4] it is at 'the check-up consultation' appointment that professional and lay meanings of attendance are at their closest, that is, the dentist knows 'something' and the patient knows 'something' of the reasons for their meeting.

In terms of professional and lay understanding both the dentist and Mrs J, in Case 2, knew 'something' as to why she had accessed care — her yearly dental visit. Mrs J attended not only in response to her knowing that she needed a scale and polish (physical) but also because she wished to look attractive for her son's wedding (psychological and social). It would seem that psycho-social impacts may play a part with regard to accessing regular care.

When a patient presents at the dental surgery as an emergency the impact of the symptoms in terms of professional and lay understanding may be at their most diverse. Dentists will expect patients to attend as soon as they become aware of their severe oral symptoms. For some patients it is not the symptom alone but rather a combination of the psycho-social impacts

Case 2

Mrs J had been a practice patient for many years and was well known to everyone in the surgery. She attended for her routine examination. On being told that she needed to see the hygienist, Mrs J responded that she had thought she needed a scale and polish and wondered if that clinical session could it be arranged to fit in, in time with her son's wedding — she wanted to 'look good' for the photographs.

together with the symptoms which provides the impetus to seek care. The example of Case 3, Mrs K and her daughter Ann, is illustrative.

The issue of translating the psycho-social impact of dental symptoms into treatment is clear in the example of Ann. Tickle *et al.*[9] suggest that it is the reporting of the physical symptom that provides the stimulus to access dental care. In Case 3 it was Ann's reporting of her 'sore mouth' together with the disruption of the household at night which provided the stimulus for mother to access care. Mother was unaware of the true state of her daughter's dentition until onset of acute symptoms. It was not physical need alone that enabled the mother to access care but the psycho-social impact of her daughter's dental symptoms.

Translating symptoms into care will be different for dentists and their patients. Professionally, dentists perceive physical symptoms as the impetus for accessing dental treatment. For patients psycho-social impacts may carry equal weight with physical discomfort and together provide the stimulus to seek dental care. The effect of this may be to distort further the

Case 3

Mrs K brought her 4-year-old daughter, Ann, to the emergency dental clinic. She thought that 'a couple of weeks ago' Ann's face had been a little red and possibly swollen but Ann had been 'out of sorts'. Mrs K had thought little of it as Ann had not complained of toothache. However for the last couple of nights Ann's sleep had been disrupted. In fact the whole household had been disturbed with Ann crying about her 'sore mouth'. Mrs K was shocked to discover that Ann had a number of decayed teeth and that one appeared abscessed. Mrs K felt that something had to be done to relieve her daughter's pain. In addition she stated 'we're all in need of a good night's sleep'.

dentist–patient interaction with regard to perceptions of professional–lay treatment need.

Professional–lay perspective 3:
Perceptions of treatment need

The concept of need reflects the difficulties inherent within the professional–lay dimension of the dentist–patient relationship. This is because need means different things to different people. A plethora of definitions of need exists.[14] These range from statements about professional assessments of health status to definitions associated with treatment procedures. In order to clarify such diversity in the definition of need three different categories have been identified. These are normative, expressed and felt need (Table 2.1). The greatest mismatch in perception of need exists in relation to unmet treatment need. It is in the need for treatment of unmet oral health needs that the professional–lay differential can have the greatest influence upon the treatment alliance.

The reasons for this are quite clear. The dental health professional's concept of need is related to his or her professional knowledge and skills and is hence connected to the patient's physical dental health status. The patient's concepts

Categorisation of treatment need

Normative need

This is professionally defined need. It is dictated by the professional training and is identified by dentists when they diagnose disease (dental caries, periodontal disease) or perceive a fall in acceptable standards of, for example, oral hygiene.

Expressed needs

Expressed needs are the needs that patients say they need both in words and actions.

Felt need

Felt need is what patients feel they need. It reflects the lay understanding and perception of dental health needs. It is what patients feel, want and think needs to be done. Patients may feel unable to talk about their wishes or may not have the words to describe their needs in this regard.

Table 2.1 Categorisation of treatment need

of need are related to psycho-social influences such as previous dental experiences and dental phobia status. The dentist's clinical skill and judgement lead to a diagnosis together with the formulation of an appropriate treatment plan. Successful treatment outcome will be dependent upon the patient's capacity to use the treatment offered. Redford and Gift[1] have stated 'before any recommended treatment can be delivered, information exchange and value negotiation must take place between dentist and patient'. The need for the dental health professional to grasp the importance of the patient's ability to understand the necessity of the treatment offered will maintain an equality within the treatment alliance and lead to a successful outcome.

In Case 4 there had been no prior discussion or information exchange with regard to referral for specialist care or maintenance programme. The scene was therefore set for a mismatch in the perception of need for periodontal treatment. The patient, Mr G, was unable to use the periodontal treatment provided by the hygienist because he had not understood the need to care for his own mouth between visits to the hygienist. The treatment alliance between Mr G and his dental health professional had been disturbed resulting in an unsuccessful treatment outcome.

Case 4

Mr G, a 35-year-old unmarried patient, had a number of deep periodontal pockets. He had been referred for periodontal care. He had now returned to the practice for maintenance therapy during which the hygienist routinely examined his mouth. However she was becoming increasingly concerned about Mr G's poor plaque control and subsequent gingivitis. Based upon her clinical experience and skill she believed that there was an unmet treatment need and began to formulate a preventive treatment plan (normative need). Mr G stated that he found it difficult to stick to the advice given to him so that he infrequently used the floss or inter-dental brushes he had been advised to buy. He felt that his gums looked 'healthy enough', 'didn't hurt' and 'were OK'. He just did not see the point to all of this. As long as his mouth looked alright and he had no pain or discomfort then he really would prefer to leave things as they were (expressed need). In fact he thought it was a waste of time and money (felt need).

Professional–lay perspective 4:
Implications for practice

It has been suggested that patients' health care and treatment needs are in fact continually changing and will be traded against other more urgent or important life needs.[15] Health needs are therefore sensitive to changes in socio-economic and/or employment status and have a tendency to vary in response to personal, family and life circumstances (psycho-social influences). Evaluating health care needs in this way connects the psycho-social impacts of dental symptoms with accessing care and with perceptions of treatment need. From a lay perspective dental symptoms affect the quality of life but psycho-social impacts also influence expressed and felt treatment needs. Therefore changes which occur in lifestyle will affect the perception of the impact of dental symptoms and treatment need. However, equivalent shifts in professional perception of treatment need may not have occurred. The dentist's perception of the patients' normative need may remain the same and hence provide a situation in which a clash occurs between the patients' changing expressed and felt needs and the professional's static

Example 1

A male patient complained that the crown on a central incisor was defective and he demanded to have it replaced. After a detailed examination the dentist agreed the crown was, to some extent, clinically defective. The old crown was removed, impressions taken and colour chosen with the patient's approval. The dentist was surprised when the patient returned some weeks after the crown had been fitted to say that it was unsatisfactory and stated it to be 'defective'. The dentist replaced the crown for a second time but the patient found it again 'defective' and requested a second opinion from a consultant. He confided to the consultant that his family circumstances had changed in that his youngest child had moved into residential care as she was severely disabled. The patient described his daughter as 'defective'. He had always hoped that his daughter would become perfect. It seemed that his wish for a perfect daughter and a perfect crown were synonymous. He remained dissatisfied with his treatment and decided to seek legal advice.

Example 2

Ms L was 28 years old when she presented. She had not been for dental treatment for many years and admitted to being 'terrified'. Many of her teeth were broken and she knew that they needed attention although they were not causing much in the way of discomfort. She felt that something had to be done before her 'front teeth went the same way'. She confided to the dentist and the dental nurse that her new partner had insisted that she have dental treatment. It was as if the option was 'visit the dentist or we finish'. By acknowledging Ms L's felt need for dental care a negotiated treatment was agreed. The treatment outcome was successful.

normative need. The result of this clash between professional and lay perspective may result in patients leaving unsatisfied with the dental care they have received.

In the two short examples above the first illustrates that when the normative need is influenced by the patient's demands for care, the patient may remain dissatisfied with the treatment outcome and consider litigation. The second case illustrates how an acknowledgement of the psycho-social influences on the patient's dental health status together with felt and expressed needs can lead to a successful treatment outcome.

Conclusions

The aim of this chapter was to present some guidance on professional and lay perspectives of the dentist–patient interaction. It would seem that a gulf may potentially exist between the way in which dental health professionals think about oral health and disease compared with their patients. It was suggested that this potential gulf may alter the dynamics of the treatment alliance. For the health professional thoughts about the impact of dental symptoms, how these are translated into accessing care and the need for dental treatment, were based upon clinical and physical dimensions of health, but this is not always so for the patient. From a lay perspective the impact of dental symptoms includes not only physical but also psychological and social dimensions. The means by which oro-facial symptoms are translated into accessing dental care and treatment need are also subjected to psycho-social influences.

Dental health professionals, by acknowledging that differences exist, will be able to maintain the equality of the dentist-patient interaction. By discussing and negotiating preventive regimes and treatment plans they will be able to provide effective dental care.

References

1. Redford M, Gift H C. Dentist-patient interactions in treatment decision-making: a qualitative study. *J Dent Educ* 1997; **61**: 16-21.
2. Weare K. The contribution of education to health promotion. In *Health Promotion: Disciplines and Diversity* R Bunton and G MacDonald (Eds). London: Routledge, 1993
3. Locker D. *An introduction to behavioural science and dentistry*. London: Routledge, 1989.
4. Coleman H, Burton J. Aspects of control on the dentist-patient relationship. *Int Soc Lang* 1985; **51**: 75-104.
5. Lamey P J, Lamb A B. Prospective study of the aetiological factors in burning mouth syndrome. *Br Med J* 1988; **296**: 1243-1246.
6. Freeman R. A psychotherapeutic approach to the understanding and treatment of a psychosomatic disorder: the case of burning mouth syndrome. In *Centres and peripheries of psychoanalysis: an introduction to psychoanalytic studies*. R Ekins and R Freeman (Eds). London: Karnac Books, 1994.
7. Leao A, Sheiham A. The development of a socio-dental measure of dental impacts on daily living. *Community Dent Health* 1996; **13**: 22-26
8. Adulyanon S, Vourapukjaru J, Sheiham A. Oral impacts affecting daily performance in a low dental disease Thai population. *Community Dent Oral Epidemiol* 1996; **24**: 385-389.

9. Tickle M, Craven R, Blinkhorn A S. An evaluation of a measure of subjective oral health status in the UK. *Community Dent Health* 1997; **13**: 175-180.

10. Ettinger R L, Jakobsen J R. A comparison of patient satisfaction and dentist evaluation of overdenture therapy. *Community Dent Oral Epidemiol* 1997; **25**: 223-227.

11. Fiske J, Davis D M, Frances C, Gelbier S. The emotional effects of tooth loss in edentulous people. *Br Dent J* 1998; 184: 90-93.

12. Freeman R. The triangle of health: applications for general practice part 1 the clinical arena. *Dent UpDate* 1997; **24**: 61-63.

13. Jacob C, Plamping D. *The practice of primary health care*. Bristol: Wright, 1989.

14. Sheiham A, Maizels J, Cushing A. New composite indicators of dental health. *Community Dent Health* 1987; **4**: 407-414.

15. Ong B N. *The practice of health services research*. London: Chapman & Hall, 1993.

The case for mother* in the surgery

The interaction of dentists with their child patients is a very special type of dentist–patient relationship. Child patients do not decide to attend on their own accord. Their mothers will often have made this decision for them. It will be mother who makes all dental health decisions for her child — when her child will be brought for dental care, decides what foods her child will eat, who will supervise tooth-brushing with a fluoride toothpaste and whether or not her child receives fluoride supplements. Mother is an integral part of dental health care for children.

Given this background, it is surprising, then, that mother is often left in the waiting room. The issue of whether the mother should or should not stay with the child during dental treatment has become a hotly debated issue in paediatric dentistry.[1] There are those who state that the accompanying adult must remain in the waiting room while others believe mother's presence in the surgery is essential. Antagonists state that the child will 'play up' in front of mother while supporters state that to separate child from mother increases anxiety and interferes with treatment compliance.[2] The latter authors suggest that the mother's presence in the surgery allows the dentist to form a relationship with mother and child which strengthens compliance, treatment and preventive regimes (the treatment alliance).[3]

Why should the debate of mother in or out of the surgery stir up such strength of feeling within the dental profession? Perhaps the answer to this question is related to the dentist's interaction with mother and child. This is a special type of dentist–patient relationship in which the dentist has to care for two people — child and mother. The dentist–patient interaction, therefore,

*The author recognises that fathers, grandparents, other relatives and/or family friends accompany children to the dentist. The noun mother will be used throughout to represent the accompanying adult.

shifts from being a two-person encounter to being a three-person encounter.[4] When mother is excluded from the surgery the dentist–child patient relationship reverts to a two-person endeavour as with adult patients. The wish to retain this familiar pattern of treatment encounter may be proposed as a reason for the exclusion of mother. Using a psychodynamic framework together with the concepts of the real relationship, the treatment alliance and transference will assist in understanding the dentist–child patient relationship and demonstrate the case for the mother being in the dental surgery during operative dental treatment.

The psychodynamic theory of the dentist–child patient relationship

Models exist[5] which help explain the dentist–child patient relationship. What is proposed here is a psychodynamic model which illustrates the quality of the interaction between dentist, child and parent during dental care. In addition this model helps in understanding the shift of feeling or attention which occurs when a dentist treats a child patient in the presence of the mother. Different aspects of the model provide appropriate explanations for this three-person endeavour, thus allowing the dentist to use it to strengthen the treatment alliance and the child's ability to accept dental care.

The real relationship

The real relationship is an equal and unique relationship between two adults. What possible relevance can it have for the dentist–child patient interaction? A real relationship does exist in the treatment of the child patient. It exists between the dentist and the parent who brings the child for care. The parent has heard about the dentist's skills with small children and it is with the parent that the equality of the interaction must be maintained. In Case 1, Jim's toothache and his emergency treatment allowed the

Case 1

Jim is a five-year-old boy. He had toothache. Father had been told that a local dentist was 'good with children' and would be willing to see a child in pain at any time. An appointment was duly arranged. On entering the surgery the dentist took father aside and obtained Jim's dental and medical history. He then turned his attention to Jim. He explained how he would numb and then extract Jim's tooth. He allowed Jim to see and touch the forceps so that Jim would understand what was happening to him. Father had been impressed by the dentist's management skills and at Jim's next appointment decided to register his two other younger children for dental care with this dentist.

real relationship between the dentist and Jim's father to be forged. This resulted in Jim's younger siblings being registered for dental treatment with the dentist. Father in this scenario acted as an advocate for Jim.

The treatment alliance
The need to reduce the child's dental anxiety is the most important aspect of managing children in the dental surgery. The intensity of the child's anxiety acts to destroy any attempt to form a treatment alliance. Everything must be done to reduce the child's anxiety so that a treatment alliance with the dentist may be achieved. The child's anticipatory and separation anxieties must be reduced. The unwanted effect of mother's own worries and concerns must be dealt with as well as the child's fears of helplessness and abandonment which arise as a result of the dental treatment itself.

The mother is an integral part of treatment of a family because she will assist the dentist to reduce the sources of anxiety which contribute to her children's fears of dental care. Although mother's personality may affect her child's ability to cope with dental care, the mother who can withstand her own anxieties together with those of her child will help the dentist to form and strengthen the treatment alliance. Irrespective of whether the child presents with pain or not, the first step in treating children is by communicating and discussing treatment options with the mother. It is in this way that mother's help is invaluable.

Anticipatory dental anxiety
The mother will be able to help her child cope with the dental experience by reducing the level of anticipatory anxiety. She should tell her child where they are going shortly before the dental appointment. The child should be encouraged to ask questions and have any questions answered. Mother must be advised to bring her child to the surgery only a few minutes before the appointment time. At the dental surgery the dentist, by using simple techniques, as tell–show–do, reduces the child's uncertainty by explaining every clinical procedure.[6] By the mother and dentist working in partnership, the child's anticipatory anxiety, whether based on previous traumatic dental experiences and/or fears of the unknown, will be reduced allowing the child to accept the treatment that is being offered.

Separation anxiety
Another source of child dental anxiety is the fear of being separated from the mother. Separation anxiety[1,7–8] is often confused with shyness in small children and it has been shown to be a good indicator of dental anxiety in childhood.[9–10] Separation anxiety must be reduced to a minimum and therefore the mother must be invited into the surgery with her child.

In Case 2, the dentist's awareness of three-year-old Jessie's separation fears together with the help of the mother assisted in building up a treatment

Case 2

Jessie arrived for her first appointment with her mother. She held tightly onto mother's hand refusing to leave her side. Jessie ignored the dentist's overtures and remained curled up on her mother's lap. With mother's agreement it was decided that Jessie would return to meet the dentist and dental nurse without any treatment being imposed upon her. Gradually over several visits Jessie left her mother's side and walked round the surgery. On one occasion she took the dentist's hand telling her that she had brought 'Dolly-dolly' who was not frightened of the dentist. Jessie climbed into the chair. At this fourth visit Jessie's teeth were examined and prophylaxis completed. Jessie had her treatment completed within several visits with her mother being present in the surgery at the time of treatment.

alliance. For several visits no dental treatment occurred as Jessie's five-minute visits deliberately coincided with lunch-time breaks. In terms of time expended it was well spent. Jessie's restorative treatment was easily completed and resulted in a number of new families being registered at the practice.

For Jessie, aged three, the degree of separation anxiety[1,8] was to be expected in a child at her stage of psychological development. For Maura, aged ten (Case 3), the inappropriateness and intensity of her separation fears were indicative of her considerable psychological difficulties.[1] Her separation anxiety was so great that she was unable to leave her mother at anytime. Mother's presence in the surgery did little to alleviate the intensity of Maura's anxieties. Indeed the extraction of an upper premolar provided the necessary stimulus to precipitate a panic attack. The intensity of the anxiety Maura experienced destroyed the treatment alliance.

Maternal dental anxiety and the treatment alliance
Difficulties in child patient management may occur when the mother is too anxious and herself too frightened of dental treatment. Although some mothers are able to contain their dental fears, there are those who experience such an intensity of anxiety that it increases their child's anxiety and disturbs the developing treatment alliance. The infectiousness of maternal anxiety is observed in children who are dentally phobic. Their mothers are themselves dentally phobic and often admit to having psychological difficulties.[11] The destruction of the treatment alliance reflects the intensity of anxiety experienced by the child which is compounded by the mother's dental anxiety status. In such cases it is better for the child to come with the

father or indeed another close relative who is less fearful and with whom the child feels comfortable and safe. This was the situation when mother accompanied Sandra (Case 4) for restorative treatment.

Case 3

Mother brought Maura to the surgery for the extraction of two upper premolar teeth for orthodontic reasons. Maura had previously coped well with dental treatment and it was decided that the teeth would be extracted immediately. After the extraction of one tooth Maura had a panic attack. She felt sick, faint and cried for mother. The intensity of the attack destroyed Maura's ability to accept any further treatment. It was decided to leave the other extraction for another time. A phone call from mother informed the dentist of Maura's psychological difficulties. As a three-year-old she had become so frightened and panicky of life in general that she had been referred to a child psychiatrist. Maura's old fears were returning. She was finding it difficult to leave her mother at any time, gradually becoming phobic of school. Mother had been so shocked by the return of Maura's anxieties that she felt that Maura would not be able to withstand the extraction of the other tooth. The intensity of Maura's panic attack had shocked both the dentist and mother. Maura was referred for secondary level hospital dental care.

Case 4

Sandra, aged nine years, was considered to be a 'good' patient being quite compliant with the dental treatment provided for her by her dentist. She had had several restorations but seemed to have taken all these in her stride. Sandra's grandmother usually brought her to the dentist and remained with her during the operative procedures. However, for Sandra's last appointment her mother also came along and like grandmother sat in the surgery. As the dentist was about to drill Sandra's tooth, mother stated nervously, 'I just hate it!' Sandra froze, became tearful and it was impossible to continue treatment. A new appointment for Sandra was made. The intervening time interval allowed the dentist to reflect upon Sandra's reaction to her mother's previous verbal outburst. A phone call ensured that grandmother would bring Sandra on her next visit. This allowed Sandra to complete her dental care.

Fears of passivity and helplessness

There is another source of anxiety which must be dealt with for the child to accept dental care. A possible source of anxiety arises from the fact that the child has to lie passively on the dental chair during treatment. This enforced passivity causes a sense of helplessness and abandonment.

The sense of helplessness in lying on a dental chair can be so intense that it interferes with the treatment alliance. It may be exacerbated by occupational anxieties arising within the dental practitioner.[12] In Case 5 the intensity of Peter's dental anxiety was such that it upset the treatment alliance. Peter's anxiety disturbed the young woman dentist who initially reacted to him in a brusque manner. Mother's interventions helped in his treatment.

The sense of helplessness and passivity must be lessened if the child is to be able to accept dental treatment. The child must be helped to turn the passive experiences of treatment into actions. For example the child can be asked to hold a face mirror so that (s)he can see what is happening inside the mouth. With other children the activity may take the form of 'playing dentist'. A small plastic mirror allows them to act the anticipated, fearful treatment experiences and this lessens helplessness and fears of abandonment.

Case 5

The young dentist could not understand Peter's anxieties and felt irritated at the thought of treating him. She had tried many times to provide dental care but Peter had always refused. This latest appointment was his 'last chance'. Otherwise he would be referred elsewhere. Despite her sense of hopelessness about caring for Peter the dentist decided to speak to his mother and this proved fruitful. Peter had been so frightened at the thought of treatment that he had not slept for the previous three nights and vomited before leaving the house. Mother had told the dentist that she had told Peter that he 'must try hard', that she would be with him during treatment. After receiving this information the dentist felt less concerned about treating Peter knowing that mother was supportive of her treatment plans. The dentist asked Peter why he was so frightened and he responded by saying, 'It was the injection'. The dentist now spent some time explaining how his gum and tooth would be numbed. Peter's mother sat beside him, encouraging him and holding her son's hand tightly when the local anaesthetic was administered. Peter was given a face mirror with the instruction to raise his hand if he wanted the dentist to stop. These simple procedures (activities) helped Peter combat his fears of passivity. With the treatment alliance restored the course of treatment was completed.

With mother's help in assisting her child 'play dentist' at home, the child's anticipatory anxiety will also be further reduced thereby strengthening the treatment alliance and the child's acceptance of dental care.[12,13]

Transference and regression

The interaction between the dentist and the adult patient is characterised by transferences and regression. The transference, for adults is a repetition of previous emotionally important relationships inappropriately (and automatically) imposed upon the person of the dentist. It is associated with regression which is reflected in a shift in the patient's attitudes. An equivalent situation does not exist in children. While children may regress in their ability to function, it is not true to say that a transference, of the type observed with adult patients, occurs in children, as the child is still attached to the mother. In children regression is more specific being related to the physical discomfort of dental treatment, pain of toothache and fears of dental treatment. The role of this regression is to reduce the child's age-adequate functioning in terms of psychological development, coping skills, cognition and motility. In other words, the child patient may be chronologically ten years old but as a consequence of regression may appear from their manner and behaviour to be much younger.

The discomfort of dental treatment as the cause of regression

Anna Freud[14] stated that any physical discomfort acts as a regressive agent in children. In the case of seven-year-old Jo, a combination of her dental anxiety together with the discomfort of having her teeth fissure sealed, resulted in regression. This was observed in her behaviour (clinging to mother), her manner (she became incommunicable) and in her motility (she was motionless). She appeared much younger than her true age.

The discomfort of dental pain as the cause of regression

Mother's discovery of her child's abscessed tooth and swollen face had been a shock to both of them (Case 6). Janet was understandably distressed by her 'sore face' and consequently clung to her mother. According to mother, Janet was an outgoing child but since she had been unwell with toothache she had not let mother out of her sight and it became clear that Janet had

---

Case 6

Janet, a four-year-old girl, arrived as an emergency patient. She clung to her mother and refused to let the dentist examine her. As the dentist put her hand up to touch Janet's swollen face, Janet started to cry.

regressed in her behaviour. Furthermore Janet was suffering with the pain of her abscessed tooth. When approached by the dentist Janet could not differentiate between the suffering caused by her dental abscess and the 'suffering' caused by the treatment to cure it.[14]

Dental anxiety as a stimulus for regression
The case of 14-year-old Nora illustrates how dental anxiety acts as a stimulus for regression (Case 7). Nora's mother always accompanied her for dental treatment and despite her considerable anxieties Nora managed to undergo any treatment required. She was nevertheless consumed with feelings of shame and humiliation, particularly when she thought about how she felt and behaved in the dental surgery, it made her feel like a baby. In this instance a false connection[15] was made between a female doctor, wearing a white coat, sitting behind Nora and the female dentist who wore a white coat, and sat behind Nora when administering dental treatment.

Case 7

The woman dentist, who treated Nora was kind and patient, encouraging her through her treatment experiences and in this regard had been helped by Nora's mother. Nora was frightened by the dentist sitting behind her. Her mother remembered that when Nora was four years old she had a general anaesthetic to have a tonsillectomy. For that operation a female anaesthetist had also sat behind Nora whilst administering the inhalation anaesthetic. This had been a traumatic experience for Nora.

Conclusions
This chapter sets out the case for the child's mother being present during treatment in the dental surgery. It illustrates how the mother is an integral part of child patient dental care. It is with the mother that the dentist forms the real relationship and it is through her that the treatment alliance between the dentist and the child is created and strengthened. For the child and dentist the mother is the greatest ally in terms of management.

References
1 Guthrie A. Separation anxiety: an overview. *Pediatr Dent* 1997; **19**: 486–490.
2 Wright G Z, Starkey P E, Gardner D E. *Parent–child separation*. In G Z Wright, P E Starkey, D E Gardner (Eds.) *Managing Children's Behaviour in the Dental Office*. St Louis: Mosby, 1983.
3 Frankl S N, Shiere F R, Fogels H R. Should the parent remain in the operatory? *ASDC J Dent Child* 1962; **29**: 150–162.

4 Kamp A A. Parent child separation during dental care: a survey of parent's preference. *Pediatr Dent* 1992; **14**: 231–235.

5 Robert J F. How important are techniques? The empathetic approach to working with children. *J Dent Child* 1995; **62**: 38–43.

6 Carson P, Freeman R. Tell-show-do: Reducing anticipatory anxiety in emergency paediatric dental patients. *Int J Health Prom Edu* 1998; 36: 87–90.

7 Blinkhorn A S. *Introduction to the dental surgery.* In R R Welbury (Ed.) Paediatric Dentistry. Oxford: Oxford University Press, 1997.

8 Bowlby J, Robertson J, Rosenbluth S. A two and half-year-old goes to the hospital. *The Psychoanal Stud Child* 1952; **7**: 82–94.

9. Holst A, Hallonsten A-L, Schroder U, Ek L, Edlund K. Prediction of behavior-management in 3-year-old children. *Scand J Dent Res* 1993; **101**: 110–114.

10 Quinonez R, Santos R G, Boyar R. Temperament and trait anxiety as predictors of child behavior prior to general anesthesia for dental surgery. *Pediatr Dent* 1997; **19**: 427–431.

11 Corkey B, Freeman R. Predictors of dental anxiety in 6 year-old children - a report of a pilot study. *ASCD J Dent* 1994: **61** ; 267–271.

12 Marcum B K, Turner C, Courts F J. Pediatric dentists' attitudes regarding parental presence during dental procedures. *Pediatr Dent* 1995; **17**: 432–436.

13 Radis F G, Wilson S, Griffen A L, Coury D L. Temperament as a predictor of behaviour during initial dental examination in children. *Pediatr Dent* 1994; **16**: 121–126.

14 Freud A. (1952) The role of bodily illness in the mental life of children. In R Ekins, R Freeman (Eds.) *The Selected Writings of Anna Freud.* Harmondsworth: Penguin Books, 1998.

15 Freeman R. A psychodynamic theory for dental phobia. *Br Dent J* 1998; **184**: 170–176.

4 The determinants of dental health attitudes and behaviours

The adoption of healthy patterns of behaviours conducive to improving and maintaining health are at the centre of health promotion strategies. Health promotion strategies based on changing care policy have been particularly successful.[1,2] However, health education programmes which have relied solely on the individual changing their own health actions have had varying levels of success[1-3].

Criticisms of these latter programmes have been directed to a lack of understanding of psycho-social factors by the health care professionals.[4] It has been suggested that providing dental health advice at the expense of understanding how health attitudes and behaviours developed, evolved and were modified with time, were cited as the main reasons for disappointing results.[5] It seemed that by ignoring the patients' life histories and experiences it was impossible to understand why patients varied so much in their reactions and responses to one-to-one dental health education.[4,5]

In an attempt to understand patients' compliance or reluctance to adhere to dental health advice, it was suggested that the development of dental health attitudes, perceptions and behaviours should be central to health education programmes.[6] It was essential that dental health professionals were acquainted with their patients' life histories. The factors, which were considered so important in the development of health attitudes and behaviours, became collectively known as the psycho-social determinants of health attitudes and behaviours.

Being aware of the psycho-social determinants of a patient's health behaviours does not give practitioners permission to blame or criticise their patients. It provides a basis for an understanding of the difficulties patients experience when complying with dental health care advice. It must be stressed that the patient does not make a conscious decision either to comply or not comply, as their ability to do so is affected by these very psycho-social determinants. Psycho-social factors intervene in the relationship with the health professional making it possible or impossible for the patient to comply. Psycho-social factors influence the treatment alliance (see Chapter 1) by reducing the means by which patients can use the information given to them for change.[4]

Dental health professionals are not immune to these psycho-social influences. Their health attitudes and behaviours are equally affected by their life experiences, including personal histories and professional training which should allow the patients' difficulties to be thought of as a dynamic interplay within the dentist-patient interaction. Indeed the dentists' own health beliefs and attitudes may influence the patients' ability to comply with the dental health message.

This chapter examines the role of psycho-social factors as determinants of health behaviours. It analyses the development of dental health attitudes and behaviours from the patient, professional and societal perspectives. The aim of this chapter is to present the practitioner with a structure with which to understand the difficulties patients may encounter when trying to comply with dental health care.

The concept of a health career

The development and evolution of health attitudes and behaviours throughout a person's life has been called a health career. A health career provides the health professional with:

> ...a description of the ways in which an individual's attitudes to a health issue develop over time.[7]

A person's health career starts at birth and so family attitudes and behaviours are the first influences upon an individual's health perceptions termed primary socialisation.[8] During childhood and adolescence health attitudes are affected by friends and peers (secondary socialisation).[8] As time passes colleagues (professionalisation)[9] and the attitudes of society (social norms) contribute to how a person perceives his/her health. Put simply, a health career describes how health perceptions are modified with time and age.[7-9]

The psycho-social determinants of health behaviours contribute to the formation of the health career but also may provide the basis for future problems which may exist when people try to change their health behaviours. When an individual attempts to modify or change their dental health behaviour the path forward is blocked by the factors which were instrumental in the construction of his/her health career in the first place. For instance the individual's socio-economic background, level of education attained, relative wealth/poverty as well as family circumstances are salient in this regard.

Previous dental health care experiences, whether good or bad, will also temper the individual's reactions to dental health education. All these psychosocial factors mould an individual's health career, and affect their readiness to modify their health attitudes and change their behaviours.

The concept of a dental health career

Dental health attitudes and behaviours develop and change with age and lifestyle as for any other aspect of health. Therefore a dental health career also exists. In truth a dental health career tracks the development of dental health attitudes from birth through adolescence to adulthood.[7]

The dental health career: Primary socialisation

In childhood the most important influences upon dental health attitudes and behaviours are those gleaned from parents and family. The small child imitates or identifies with the parents' attitudes and behaviours. During these early years the child mimics the parents' actions. The parent, by caring for the child's bodily and dental health, shows and teaches the young child how to take care of herself.[10]

It is important to emphasise that small children do not necessarily want their faces washed or teeth cleaned and the parent must do this for them.[10] Gradually, as the child's manual dexterity develops, the child will brush her teeth and wash her face as it was done previously by the parent. It is through this process of emotional identification[8] with the parent, a process which has been called 'primary socialisation', that children learn to take care of their bodies and teeth.

Case 1

By way of illustration of the process of primary socialisation, a female patient's experiences with her 15-month-old daughter are characteristic. The mother had always cleaned her daughter's teeth and this had become quite a game at bed-time until her daughter insisted on 'doing it herself'. She held the brush tight, pushing it into her own mouth, thus imitating her mother's own actions and thus learning how to care for her teeth.

The dental health career: Secondary socialisation

As time progresses the child will start school. At school other influences — teachers and friends and so forth — will shape the child's dental health attitudes and behaviours. As the child makes attachments outside the family — with parental substitutes such as teachers and peers — another, similar process of emotional identification occurs.[8] Through the process known as 'secondary socialisation' the child emulates the attitudes and behaviours of friends and teachers. Occasionally this may lead to difficulties with differences in health attitudes and behaviours between home and school, resulting in what is called 'culture clash'. This culture clash has been reported to occur when dental health professionals' children attend school. Case 2 is typical of such experiences encountered by dental health professionals.

Case 2

Mrs P, a dental health promotion officer, complained about the school her son was attending. The teaching was excellent and she was delighted with the care afforded to her boy but during the last few days at school her son, like the other children, had been given a sweet as a reward for his excellent behaviour. Mrs P, personally, restricted her son's confectionery eating to a Saturday. She felt that he was receiving 'mixed messages' from home and school as a result of the school's reward system.

The importance of school based health education, nevertheless, has been recognised as a means of helping children develop their own health care attitudes and behaviours. The importance placed upon peers as advocates in this regard has been successfully used in child-to-child teaching programmes.[11] These programmes recognise the value of peers as a means of providing dental health information to other, usually younger children. In the peer group teaching scenario the older child not only gains a greater understanding of the needs of younger children but also develops his/her own dental health care skills

As time progresses the child enters pre-adolescence and adolescence.[12] During pre-adolescence and adolescence more and more friendships are made with people outside the home. The shift from parents and family to friends and peers is mirrored by a change in dental health care attitudes and behaviours. Difficulties arise when the adolescent's wishes are opposed by those of the parent. Recent research examining non-compliance with orthodontic care has clearly shown that it is the conflict between parent and adolescent which influences the success of continuing orthodontic treatment.[13]

Case 3 illustrates how conflict between a mother and her son affected compliance. What can be learnt from Ms H's experience with Keith? First, Keith had not chosen to return to complete his orthodontic treatment — that had

Case 3

The dentist, Ms H, was asked to see Keith, a 14-year-old boy, for orthodontic care. Keith already had experience of orthodontic treatment which had failed. Mother was very keen for Keith to have orthodontic treatment and for it to be a success. He had been told by mother that following the initial treatment failure he was now being given a second chance. On examination it was apparent that he had not cleaned his teeth for some days. Ms H referred him to her hygienist and it was decided that before orthodontic treatment would begin Keith would need to improve his oral hygiene. The overall treatment was explained to him, including the need for two further tooth extractions. At this news Keith looked worried and in the ensuing weeks Keith's oral hygiene gradually became worse. Ms H was furious. When Ms H discussed Keith's deteriorating gum health with him, Keith mentioned that his mother nagged him about brushing his teeth. Ms H stated that she felt that Keith was 'a hopeless case'.

been mother's decision. Secondly, he was dentally anxious and he worried about the prospect of having more teeth extracted. Thirdly, he had made a transference to Ms H, whom he felt was like his mother 'nagging [him]' and finally, in terms of his psychological development was still not interested in his appearance (pre-adolescence). These four psycho-social factors, recognisable by Keith's behaviour and demeanour, contributed to his non-compliance. In later discussion with Ms H, he admitted that he felt that the treatment was being foisted upon him and therefore had decided not to be co-operative. In protest Keith had refused to clean his teeth.

The dental health career: Tertiary socialisation[7–9]

In adulthood, psycho-social factors serve to sustain a pressure on individuals which affect their dental health. The process by which this occurs has been termed 'tertiary socialisation'. Tertiary socialisation does not necessarily occur in the natural order of things, but may be imposed upon the individual by outside agencies. It is proposed that three aspects of tertiary socialisation exist. The first of these is associated with dental health education, the second with the process of professionalisation and the third with the influence of social norms. Tertiary socialisation may (as in professionalisation) or may not (as in dental health education) involve an identification with another person (parent, peer or colleague) or group of people (society) and may or may not be associated with a power differential between people or groups within society. In these respects tertiary socialisation may differ from either primary or secondary socialisation.

Tertiary socialisation and dental health education[7,8]
When the aim of tertiary socialisation in the guise of dental health education claims to modify health attitudes and change behaviours, it is doomed to failure. Health education, given in this context, takes little or no account of the psycho-social factors which contributed to inappropriate health actions in the first place. Some people, as in the case of Mr G (see Chapter 2), may feel there is little point in modifying or changing their dental health behaviours. In such instances there may be a reinstatement of previous behaviours which were detrimental to the patient's dental health. In other circumstances competing lifestyle and health priorities may contribute to the patient's health decisions and actions. The issue of smoking cessation in combination with the prevention of dental caries are examples of how competing health priorities may result in apparent non-compliance.

Mr T could have proved to be a difficult case — his compliance with his doctor's advice competing with that of his dentist's. In order to help Mr T in his conflict — whose advice to take — the hygienist had to acknowledge the need to find yet another substitute for his cigarettes. She suggested the use of sugar-free chewing gum or sugar-free sweets. By discovering the reason for Mr T's apparent non-compliance the hygienist was able to find a solution to enable him to maintain his behaviour change. Mr T, however, was exceptional as he was determined to change. He was able to use the advice given to him to modify and maintain his new and healthier pattern of behaviour.

Case 4

Mr T attended his dentist on a regular basis. His dental health status remained stable and apart from the occasional scale and polish nothing remarkable, in terms of his dental health status, was noted although he was a smoker. It was with some surprise that, at his next annual examination, a number of carious lesions was detected. Mr T was referred to the practice hygienist to discover why he had developed so many carious lesions. He did not describe himself as a heavy smoker but had felt that 'the time had come to give up'. He had been told that 'keeping [his] mouth occupied would help him break the habit'. Every time he craved a cigarette he popped a boiled sweet into his mouth. He reckoned he was eating a lot of sweets.

Tertiary socialisation and professionalisation[9]

As mentioned previously, professionalisation, (see Chapter 2), is the process by which an individual becomes a member of a professional body.[9] Professionalisation is characterised by a shift from lay to professional health agendas thereby modifying communication styles (this will be covered in Chapter 7) and changes in health attitudes and behaviour.

With regard to transformation of health care regimes, three processes are important. First, there is the process of identifying with other dental health professionals. As with secondary socialisation, the admired teacher or colleague will be emulated. Teachers' and colleagues' dental health attitudes, clinical and personal actions will be incorporated into the student's patterns of behaviour. These will be observed and incorporated into the acquisition of new skills and knowledge.

The second process in professionalisation is connected with acquiring new health information. Therefore, transformations in health attitudes are also related to an increased awareness of the aetiology of oral diseases. Examples of changing patterns of health care are to be found in the oral hygiene regimes of pre-clinical dental students. When asked how many used dental floss, few replied in the affirmative. The same students, a year later, had changed their behaviour as the majority were now using floss on a daily basis.

These shifts in behaviour were associated with modifications in attitude. For dental students a change in health attitude was associated with a concern for their gingival health. Thinking in this way allows the role of a disease orientated approach to be acknowledged in their preventive health care. This suggests that the changes observed in health actions are, in part, a result of a heightened awareness of the pathological process. As an example (Case 5) concern about personal gingival health was raised by an hygienist student.

Although acquired early in the practitioner's professional life these shifts in health attitudes and behaviour have a long-term stability. For instance, dentists' children have lower experiences of dental caries compared with equivalent professional groups. These findings suggest that the changes in personal health actions acquired during professionalisation remain fixed with time.[14]

Case 5

During an oral examination, the dentist commented that the student hygienist had a localised area of gingivitis. The young woman became upset and stated, 'This is dreadful! Gingivitis in my mouth, where is it! I must see! It must be attended to immediately, I can't be brushing properly.'

The third process associated with professionalisation affects society at large. It does this through its power and influence. The power is also connected to the knowledge and training on which the work of the profession is based. Dentistry has gained a monopoly over an area of expertise and the right to self-determination. The recognition of this expertise and knowledge by society affords members of the profession a place within society which influences their dental health attitudes and behaviour.

Tertiary socialisation and social norms
Societal attitudes or social norms affect attitudes towards dental health. At a society level, for instance, public attitudes towards water fluoridation has effectively reduced the availability of fluoride in the public water supplies.

Social norms can be considered as expressions of the beliefs and attitudes of people who belong to a particular social group. In this sense social norms not only afford a cohesiveness to the group but also permit it to have a sense of identity. It is this identity which gives the group its characteristics. Dental health promotion strategies which are targeted at groups of people, in what has been termed the settings approach, acknowledges the importance of social norms as a salient element in behaviour change.

It has been suggested that social norms have a tenacity of their own. Nevertheless, they may be gradually modified with time and between generations or change abruptly with social mobility. For example, social norms can be gradually modified within a three generation family with the attitudes of grandparents being quite different to those of their grandchildren. Social mobility, in terms of movement through socio-economic groups, has been shown to affect dental health attitudes and behaviour in an abrupt way. Social mobility via marriage has been shown to provide the impetus for changes in dental health care actions being associated with changing social norms.[15]

Conclusions
It has been proposed that people's attitudes and behaviours towards health in general and dental health in particular, are a culmination of life experiences and events. Influences from childhood, through school and into adulthood have been shown to determine an individual's health perceptions. This has been called a 'health career'. Understanding how health behaviours evolve, develop and are modified with time, allows dental health professionals to take a first step in appreciating the complexities involved when people attempt to modify their dental health care attitudes and behaviour.

References
1 Downie R S, Fyfe C, Tannahill A. *Health promotion, models and values.* Oxford: Oxford Medical Publications, 1995

2 Health Education Authority. *Effectiveness of oral health promotion: a review.* Summary Bulletin 7; London: Health Education Authority 1997.

3 Kay E J. Locker D. Is dental health education effective? A systematic review of current evidence. *Community Dent Oral Epid* 1996; **24**: 231–235

4 Gift H C. *Social factors in oral health promotion.* In Oral Health Promotion (Eds. L Schou, A S Blinkhorn): Oxford: Oxford University Press, 1993.

5 French J. Boundaries and horizons: the role of health education within health promotion. *Health Edu J* 1990; **94**: 7–10.

6 Blinkhorn A S. Evaluating and planning of oral health promotion programmes. In *Oral Health Promotion* (Eds. L Schou, A S Blinkhorn): Oxford: Oxford University Press, 1993.

7 Weare K. *The contribution of education to health promotion.* In Health Promotion: Disciplines and Diversity (Eds R Bunton and G MacDonald). London: Routledge, 1993

8. Baric L. Social expectations versus personal preferences — two ways of influencing health behaviour. *J Inst H Edu* 1977; **15**: 23–27

9. Locker D. *An introduction to behavioural science and dentistry.* London, Routledge 1989

10 Freud A. The role of bodily illness in the mental life of children. In *The Selected Anna Freud* (Eds. R Ekins, R Freeman) Harmondsworth: Penguin Books, 1998.

11 Bunting G. *Promoting dental health in schools: a child-to-child approach.* Belfast: The Queen's University of Belfast, 1997. Unpublished MPhil Thesis.

12 Freud A. On certain difficulties in the preadolescent's relation to his parents. In *The Selected Anna Freud* (Eds. R Ekins, R Freeman) Harmondsworth: Penguin Books, 1998.

13 Pratelli P. *Orthodontic treatment: parents' perceptions, attitudes and knowledge.* London: University of London, 1998. Unpublished PhD Thesis.

14 McDonald S, Sheiham S, Cowell C. Methods of preventing dental caries used by dentists for their own children. *Br Dent J* 1981; **151**: 118–121

15 Beal J F, Dickson S. Dental attitudes and behaviour related to vertical social mobility by marriage. *Community Dent Oral Epid* 1975; **3**: 174–178.

Barriers to accessing and accepting dental care

Dental health professionals often experience difficulties when they try to help their patients acquire and maintain actions which are conducive to preserving their dental health. Nevertheless despite repeated attempts there may be no change in the patient's behaviour and indeed occasionally some patients may seem to deteriorate rather than improve. The patient may feel criticised while the dentist may feel there is little point in continuing. Feelings of hopelessness and despondency colour the dentist–patient interaction with the patient being thought of as impossible and non-compliant.

The patients' behaviour, however, is only one aspect of the non-compliant story. The other parts of this tale are to be found in the patients' life experiences and personal histories. The difficulties patients experience when trying to comply with dental health advice are not conjured up for the here and now but have their roots in earlier times. For instance, they may be associated with the era in which the patient grew up or with how highly their family rated dental health care amongst other competing lifestyle priorities, or perhaps they were related to previous unfortunate dental health care experiences. All of these factors would affect the patients' feelings, beliefs and attitudes with regard to complying with dental health care.

These are the psycho-social determinants of dental health attitudes and behaviour. They not only form the kernel and impetus for an individual to adopt a particular dental health action, but they may also provide the basis for the formation of obstacles to accepting and accessing dental health care. In this way it may be proposed that these psycho-social factors could be likened to 'a knife that cuts both ways'. On the one hand they may allow the patient to modify or change their dental health actions, while on the other, they may act as obstructions which seem to block any modification in health behaviour.

In order to examine the role of psycho-social factors as obstacles or barriers to behaviour change, one dental health care action that could be considered by way of illustration is dental attendance. By thinking about dental attendance as a health care action, it is evident that three perspectives must be considered. These are from the patient's perspective, the professional's perspective and that of society.[1] It is beyond the remit of this chapter to discuss societal barriers of dental attendance other than to state that they exist.

It is the aim of this chapter, to describe what is meant by barriers to accessing and accepting dental health care. Examining the content of these barriers allows the dental health professional to take the next step in understanding their patients' difficulties when complying with dental health advice.

Psycho-social factors as barriers to accessing dental health care

When considering the need for regular dental attendance, it is apparent that there is a discord which exists within the profession. While there has been little dispute with regard to the role of sugars in caries, the importance of fluoride use in the prevention of dental caries and the removal of plaque in the promotion of periodontal health, the same cannot be said for the regular dental examination. Argument and debate concerning the appropriateness and effectiveness of regular dental attendance have captured the minds of the profession and public alike. Concerns about the effect of regular dental attendance upon oral health has resulted in a number of opinions ranging from those who perceived it as a integral part of peoples' health behaviours,[2,3] to those who viewed it as dental hegemony.[4,5] Irrespective of the rights or wrongs of the debate, the fact remains that some people are unable to attend for dental care on a regular or routine basis.[6,7] The reasons for their inability to access care in the usual way need to be answered.

From the 1980s through to the 1990s[8,9] studies were conducted to find out why this state of affairs existed. The word barrier replaced the word obstacle and was coined as a means of conceptualising the difficulties people experienced when accessing dental care. Nevertheless it led to the idea that one factor relating to access to dental care could be thought of in physical terms. For some patients, physical problems did arise (for example, managing stairs) when trying to gain access to the dental surgery. For some dentists physical barriers existed with regard to the inequity of services. While, within society as a whole, insufficient political support for health care funding could influence availability of dental services.

To think of barriers as mere physical structures barring the patient's way for treatment, excludes the role of psycho-social factors as obstacles to dental attendance.[4] In this respect, psycho-social factors acquired a passive connotation rather than in their usual guise as active components associated with developing and evolving health attitudes and behaviours. Barriers to dental health care could now be considered as static factors which reduced the patient's entry to the dental surgery and treatment. In this way psycho-social factors provided a framework around which dental health professionals could plan their strategies to develop and maintain accessible dental practices for their patients.[1]

The Federation Dentaire Internationale[1] (FDI) suggested that three separate category of barrier should be considered. The first of these related specifically to the individual and included:

Lack of perceived need, anxiety and fear, financial considerations and lack of access.

The second category related to the dental profession. They included:

Inappropriate manpower resources, uneven geographical distribution, training inappropriate to changing needs and demands and insufficient sensitivity to patient's attitudes and needs.

The third and final category of barrier related to society:

Insufficient public support of attitudes conducive to health, inadequate oral health care facilities, inadequate oral health manpower planning and insufficient support for research.

Within the two-person encounter, which is the dentist–patient relationship, the psycho-social aspects of the barriers to the receipt of dental attendance are particularly important. Attitudes, concerns and financial responsibilities act as barriers with regard to accessing (the patient) and providing (the dentist) dental care. For society as a whole, norms in relation to the importance of dental health care affect regularity of dental attendance.[10]

If practitioners are to care for patients with special treatment needs it was necessary to consider how psycho-social factors[11] influence the patients' ability to access dental care, how the dental health professional's concerns about practice viability affect treatment choices and referral patterns[12] and how societal influences[10] affect access to dental health care.

The FDI classification of barriers reflects their psycho-social composition. Thinking in this way provides the means by which barriers to accessing dental care could be understood, first from the patient's and, secondly, from the dental health professional's points of view. This gives practitioners an increasing understanding of the difficulties they and their patients may experience when they, respectively, provide and access dental care.

Resistances as barriers to accepting dental health care

Another more flexible or dynamic view of barriers to dental health care exists and these have been referred to as resistances.[13] Resistances are said to exist within the dentist–patient relationship and are subject to changes in intensity. Resistances can therefore strengthen or weaken the treatment alliance. Essentially they may act to prevent the patient from progressing from accessing care to accepting dental treatment.

It is proposed that to understand the concept of barriers to accessing and accepting dental care these two models must be considered. The first is the psycho-social model. It provides a means by which practitioners can formulate policy to allow them to develop and maintain accessible general practices. The second is a psychodynamic model based upon the concept of the resistances. By understanding this concept, dentists will be able to appreciate the difficulties their patients experience when accepting dental care. By acknowledging the presence of resistances, they will be able to strengthen the treatment alliance. An awareness of the psychodynamic model of barriers to dental care provides the dental health professional with an appreciation of what barriers mean for their patients and the dentist–patient interaction.

When the patient has accessed dental care (s)he must make a decision about accepting the suggested treatment. It would seem that at this point in the dentist–patient interaction the quality and character of the barrier has changed. It can now be thought of as a dynamic force opposing the forward progression from accessing care to dental treatment. In this way barriers are conceptualised as 'resistances'. Resistances are not static obstructions but ebb and flow in accordance with the patient's feelings, worries and anxieties, on the one hand, and the desire for treatment on the other. The dynamic character of the resistances permits them to use any fears, concerns, difficult circumstances or situations that patients may experience to prevent them from accepting dental treatment. In other words any tactic will be used to prevent accessing care and hence cause a delay in treatment. Adults, for instance, may use the opportunity of a sudden upsurge at work to cancel an appointment or may just simply forget to come to the surgery at the appointed time. The case of Mrs M is illustrative (Case 1) in this regard in that by forgetting to bring her partial denture to the surgery she delayed the date of a feared extraction.

However to present the view that the resistances are all powerful and destructive would be to ignore the patient's wishes for dental treatment. It is not that the patient does not realise that the dentist is there to help or that the patient does not wish to have the treatment, it is that his fear counteracts this wish and prevents the forward movement to accepting regular dental care. To enable the forward progression from accessing care to accepting treatment the patient must be able to allow that part of herself that wishes for care to

Case 1

Mrs M was 35 years old and as a result of an accident needed the extraction of her upper, right, central incisor. It was decided that she would have an addition to her spare partial denture so that it could be worn immediately after the extraction. An appointment was made for impressions. Mrs M arrived but had left her denture at home. Although Mrs M had seemed to accept the need for the extraction of her upper central incisor her actions (leaving the denture at home) betrayed her true feelings. A resistance based upon her fears of how she would look after the extraction was the basis of forgetting her spare partial denture. Treatment had been delayed.

outweigh the resistances (the worries, fears and anxieties). The following is a common place observation and illustrates the patient's indecision or conflict in this regard:

> A man who has gone to the dentist because of an unbearable toothache will nevertheless try to hold the dentist back when he approaches the sick tooth with a pair of forceps.[13]

In the above the man's fears of the extraction (the resistance) were nearly enough to prevent the extraction of the 'sick tooth'. The resistances are barriers which need to be got over. Some patients, irrespective of the difficulties encountered, overcome their resistances and attend for dental treatment. This was the case for Mrs L (Case 2) who despite having to organise child care for the afternoon of the appointment still managed to be at the surgery at the appointed time.

Case 2

Mrs L ran into the surgery, fearful that she was late. She told the receptionist that there had been a mix up with her child care. Her mother who lived close by was to mind the children for her but she was sick. This meant contacting her mother-in-law who lives two bus journeys from her home, getting the children ready and then getting the two buses back to the surgery — she was whacked! She was looking forward to the rest in the chair before her return trip.

Resistances in children are contemporaneous with the stage of the child's personality development. The child's behaviour will betray his thoughts, worries and feelings about dental treatment (Case 3).

Case 3

An amusing example of some children's ingenuity in order to avoid a visit to the dentist is illustrated by Tim, aged 8. His mother had asked an aunt, who did not live in the town, to pick Tim up from school and take him to the dentist. Mother reassured the aunt that Tim knew the exact location of the surgery as he had been there on many occasions. The surgery was in fact sited in the street next to the school. Tim was collected at the agreed time. He told his aunt that he was not sure as to the correct location of the dentist and he would have to search for it. He walked his aunt around and around the neighbourhood for 30 minutes. Suddenly, as if by magic, Tim came upon the surgery. He was now too late for the appointment and had effectively delayed treatment to another time.

Other children will delay the start of treatment by talking incessantly. Another clinical situation exists with young children. Young children who cannot differentiate between the pain caused by the suffering of their sore teeth and that caused by treatment, or those with learning difficulties who may not understand what is happening,[14] may refuse dental treatment. In conjunction with mother's agreement the best course of action may be to facilitate referral to secondary level care. Such was the situation for Diane, aged 11, who had learning difficulties:

Case 4

Diane's dentist was fond of her but had failed in his attempts to enable Diane to accept the dental care he was trying to provide. Diane could just about tolerate a mirror in her mouth. Diane's verbal capacity was poor and she was unable to tell the dentist how she felt. It was apparent that the dentist's attempts to enable Diane to accept care had failed and in agreement with her mother it was decided to refer Diane for specialist dental care.

Dental attendance patterns may also be upset during adolescence. Adolescents who perceive the dental health professional as yet another parental figure imposing their will upon them, may miss scheduled appointments. These actions are indications that resistances are at work and should alert the dentist that all is not well. The patients' actions will provide the practitioner with the means to counteract the effect of the resistances and hence strengthen the treatment alliance (see Chapters 1 and 3). Observing the patients' behaviour and actions may prevent them from erecting barriers and missing scheduled appointments.

Resistance is a dynamic way of conceptualising barriers which exist and prevent the progression from accessing to accepting dental care. The resistances use any means available to form a barrier to prevent the patient accepting dental care. In this way they may become the practitioner's greatest enemy. However as patients' actions and behaviours betray their true feelings about the proposed treatment, resistances may become the dentist's greatest support. The recognition of resistances in the form, for example, of forgetting, alerts the dentist to the patient's concerns about treatment. Discussing a patient's worries allows the dental health professional to strengthen the treatment alliance by formulating and negotiating treatment plans with which the patient is able to comply.

The acceptance of treatment plans includes compliance with preventative regimes. Therefore an understanding of the resistances within the dentist–patient interaction allows the dental health professional to appreciate the patient's ambivalence when attempting to change his health behaviours (see Chapter 9).

Conclusions

It has been suggested that barriers to dental health are the passive aspect of the psycho-social determinants of health attitudes and behaviours. These factors may assist in behaviour modification or act to prevent any forward movement to accessing or accepting health care advice.

One specific dental health action was considered — regular dental attendance. It was clear at the outset that an obstacle existed at a professional level since dentistry itself was divided with regard to the appropriateness of regular dental attendance. Nevertheless since the 1980s, the work by Finch and colleagues[8] on the barriers to accessing regular dental care has led to an examination of the factors used by patients and dentists alike to inhibit and reduce access to dental health care.

The idea that barriers were erected not only as a result of the patients' psycho-social background but also as a consequence of professional attitudes and characteristics was voiced by the FDI[1]. This suggested that as the dentist–patient interaction was a two-person endeavour, barriers must also be considered within a two-person framework. It would be within this two-person framework that barriers to accessing and accepting dental care could be conceptualised.

It has been proposed, that barriers of a different character or quality exist in relation to accepting dental treatment. Barriers to accessing and accepting dental care are the same but possess different characteristics or qualities. First, there are those which are psycho-social in their character and are related to accessing dental care. Second there are those which are more dynamic and act within the dentist–patient relationship. These latter barriers or resistances, which may or may not also include psycho-social factors (for example, dental anxiety), reduce the patient's ability to accept dental care thereby weakening the treatment alliance.

It is by an appreciation of the character of the barriers to first accessing and second accepting dental care that dental health professionals can help their patients adopt behaviours conducive to oral health.

References

1 Cohen L K. Converting unmet need for care to effective demand. *Int Dent J* 1987; **37**: 114–116.
2 Elderton R J. Routine six-monthly checks for dental disease ? *Br Dent J* 1985; **159**: 277–278.
3 Levine R S. *The scientific basis of dental health education. A Policy Document* (4th edition). London: Health Education Authority, 1996.
4 Illich I. *Limits to medicine. medical nemesis: the expropriation of health.* Harmonsworth: Penguin Books, 1976.
5 Sheiham A. Is there a scientific basis for the six-monthly dental examinations? *Lancet* 1977; **2**: 442–444.
6 Todd J E, Lader D. *Adult dental health 1978 United Kingdom.* London: HMSO, 1981.
7 Todd J E, Lader D. *Adult dental health 1988 United Kingdom.* London: HMSO, 1991.
8 Finch H, Keegan J, Ward K. *Barriers to the receipt of dental care - a qualitative research study.* London: Social and Community Planning Research, 1988.
9 Adams E K, Freeman R, Gelbier S, Gibson B J. Accessing primary dental care in three inner city boroughs. *Comm Dent Health* 1997; **14**: 108–112.
10 Hendricks S, Freeman R, Sheiham A. Why inner city mothers take their pre-school children for medical and dental check-ups. *Community Dent Health* 1990; 7: 33–42.
11 Gift H C. *Social factors in oral health promotion.* In Oral Health Promotion (Eds. L Schou, AS Blinkhorn) Oxford: Oxford University Press, 1993.
12 Gibson B J, Freeman R. Dentists practising in Lothian Treat HIV-Seropositive Patients: Is This A Resolution Of Conflict Or A Case of Hobson's Choice? *Br Dent J* 1996; **180**: 34–37.
13 Freud S. (1917) Resistances and repression. In *Introductory Lectures on Psychoanalysis.* Harmondsworth: Penguin Books, 1976.
14 Freud A.(1952) The role of bodily illness in the mental life of children. In *The Selected Anna Freud* (Eds. R Ekins, R Freeman) Harmondsworth: Penguin Books, 1998.

Barriers to accessing dental care: patient factors

The idea that barriers to accessing and accepting dental care were related to psycho-social factors, which could be explained as resistances, has been previously considered (see Chapter 5). It was proposed that barriers to accessing and accepting dental care could be thought of within a two-person framework which reflected the dentist–patient relationship. It was further suggested that there was a need to examine the sources of the barriers themselves, from both patient and practitioner perspective (see Chapter 7), since, by doing so would allow a greater understanding of patient compliance and the role of the dentist with regard to providing accessible dental care. The purpose of this chapter is to examine the role of barriers from the patient point of view.

The source of the barriers that patients' experience in relation to accessing dental care are said to arise as a result of their life experiences and psycho-social background. These psycho-social factors are thought to provide the environment which help or hinder patients accessing care. In the dental literature, lists of psycho-social factors are given to explain patients' avoidance of dental care and to provide reasons for non-compliance with treatment and preventive regimes. These factors are said to include socio-economic status, age, gender, ethnicity, perception of need, dental anxiety states, feelings of vulnerability and so forth.[1-3] From this list of factors four main groups of barriers[2] have been identified. These are dental anxiety, financial costs, perceptions of need and lack of access.

With such a plethora of psycho-social factors acting as barriers what remains important is to consider how they influence dental attendance and affect compliance with treatment and preventive regimes. It is proposed that psycho-social factors do not act independently of each other but combine to act in unison. It is the quantitative nature of their combination which reduces access to care, resulting in non-attendance and non-compliance. For example, lifestyle commitments together with dental anxiety, may combine and form a barrier which hinders access to care. The division, therefore, of psycho-social factors into individual barriers may be, in this regard, artificial. Nevertheless, using a psycho-social structure allows the patient's dental attendance and compliance with preventive regimes to be understood.

Psycho-social factors as barriers to accessing dental care

Dental anxiety states

Dental anxiety[4,5] has been highlighted as being one of the most important barriers with regard to dental attendance. There is the view that anyone who presents with fear of dental treatment experiences an equivalent intensity of emotion or affect which results in the avoidance of dental care. However, despite their considerable dental fears some patients accept regular dental treatment.[6] It would seem that the relationship between dental anxiety and avoidance is not a simple one. Depending on the intensity of anxiety experienced, the fearful patient may find dental treatment troublesome or look upon it as an intolerable encounter.

How can such clinical observations be understood? The answer lies in defining what is meant by dental phobia* and differentiating it from dental anxiety. The diagnosis of dental phobia cannot be made solely on the basis of the presenting complaint (the patient's anxiety state) but only in conjunction with the patient's previous dental attendance history. The patient who experiences a high intensity of anxiety together with a history of avoiding dental care invites a diagnosis of dental phobia to be made. It is for these patients that fear and anxiety acts as a barrier to accessing and accepting regular dental care.

The distinction between dental anxiety and dental phobia is important. It provides the dental health professional with the means of assessing the likelihood of success with the fearful patient. For instance, the patient with high dental anxiety whose anticipatory fears can be ventilated may be successfully treated.[7] The dentally phobic patient's anxiety will destroy the treatment alliance (see Chapter 1) rendering dental care impossible. Thus the dental phobic will remain an irregular dental attender.

Dental health professionals must be able to identify patients who have special psychological needs. The use of psychological questionnaires such as the Dental Anxiety Scale[8] or the Modified Dental Anxiety Scale[9] may be helpful in identifying such individuals. These simple questionnaires are short, quick, easy to complete and the user is provided with cut off scores

*A phobia is an irrational fear of a place or an object with avoidance of that place or object.

above which a patient may be designated as being dental phobic. When they are used in conjunction with questions relating to the patients' dental history, the dentist will be in a position to identify the patient who has psychological special needs. In this way the dentist will be in a position to assist the dentally anxious or dentally phobic patient access dental health care.

As a barrier to accessing dental care, dental anxiety in children may be a consequence of the child's stage of personality development, parental dental anxieties or the parent's fears and wishes to deny her child any distress or anxiety. This wish may be a culmination of mother's own anxieties together with her disquiet at the sight of her child's distress and unhappiness. Such difficulties on the parent's behalf may result in the parent delaying care. Only when an emergency situation arises can the parent bear to subject the child to treatment. The following two vignettes are illustrative. Both of the boys, mentioned below, were aged 8 and had experience of extractions under general anaesthetic. Both returned for a prophylaxis and discussion of future preventive and restorative treatments. However, whereas Paul's mother readily accepted her child's anxieties, Rob's mother, because of her own fears and concerns for her child's well-being, denied their existence. This resulted in Paul (Case 1) managing his worries and Rob (Case 2) being treated, with difficulty.

Case 1

Paul was worried about going to the dentist as he had had four molars extracted at the previous visit. Paul was sure that the dentist would take out all of his teeth and told mother so. Recognising her son's dental anxiety she reassured him that this appointment was to clean his teeth. Paul was able to contain his worries and lay quietly to have his teeth polished.

Case 2

Rob had a similar dental experience to Paul. However at his appointment he wriggled about in the chair, hardly being able to open his mouth. With difficulty his teeth were polished. When his mother was asked if Rob was nervous she stated, 'No, he's not frightened, he likes coming to the dentist'. Mother's own dental anxiety together with the denial of her son's dental fear culminated in Rob's difficulty in accepting dental care.

The need for the dental health professional to be able to identify children who are dentally anxious has been shown to be of great importance. Prior knowledge of the dentally anxious child can help the dentist improve dental treatment experiences, thereby reducing the potency of dental anxiety as a barrier to accessing dental care.

As with adults, psychological questionnaires have been developed which have been shown to be of value when assessing children's dental anxiety. Assessments of child dental anxiety include pictorial representations[9] of the dental situation as well as asking the child how they feel about items of dental treatment such as the injection or the drill.[10]

Concerns that asking children about dental worries will increase their fears and anxieties have not been substantiated. In fact prior information in 'tell–show–do' scenarios have been shown to reduce child anticipatory dental anxieties and hence barriers to dental attendance.[11]

Financial costs

Financial costs of dental treatment remain a significant barrier to accessing dental care.[4,5] Statistics throughout the world show that peoples' ability to access regular dental care is directly related to their annual income. Interestingly the effect of annual income influences the entire family's dental attendance patterns. Children living in areas of social deprivation are, for instance, less likely to attend for restorative care; their irregular pattern of dental attendance mirroring that of their parents.[12] When affordability of dental care is combined with socio-economic status (SES), it appears that those from lower SES access care less often and admit to being less satisfied with treatment they received compared with others.

Dissatisfaction with dental treatment may be illustrated by the case of Jean, aged 23. She was on income support. Jean was disappointed with the colour and appearance of veneers which had been fitted to her upper incisor teeth. She confided in the nurse, 'If I was paying for these he'd change them … he won't do it … 'cause I get them for free'.

The difficulties and problems encountered by people on low income is said to be related to the degree of competition for the families' disposable income. Where competition is the greatest, dental treatment may be felt as an unaffordable luxury and, while being valued, may be low on a list of priorities when compared with other essential commodities. Ideas such as these suggest that an inverse care law is operative with those in greatest need receiving the least in the way of dental health care.[12]

Perceptions of need

Peoples' perceptions of treatment need range from those who attend on a regular basis with no visible sign of normative need to those who attend only when in pain. Patients' responses[13] when invited to attend for a routine examination, appear to be influenced by dental anxiety status, previous dental experiences and lifestyle commitments. Patients' perceptions of treatment need are under the control of the psycho-social determinants of dental health. Hence the impetus to change felt need into demand for care (see Chapter 2) is thought to be based upon a combination of psycho-social factors.

The idea that psycho-social factors can help (enable) or hinder (inhibit) access to regular dental care by influencing perception of need may be illustrated by examining demographic variables. For instance, people from a higher SES rather than a lower SES,[4,5] women rather than men, younger rather than older, those with greater access to private rather than public transport, all seem to attend more regularly for dental care.

For those with busy lifestyles there is the tendency to use emergency services or delay dental treatment. Time urgency was given as the reason for attending an emergency clinic by Mr J, a long distance lorry driver. He felt that regular dental attendance was a good idea but his job made it impossible for him. He felt it would be wrong to make and break appointments and so opted for emergency care:

'You come here, you have to wait a bit — but that's OK ... fits in with my job better ... they'll take the tooth out, fill it whatever and then I'll be back at work this afternoon.'

Time urgency as a barrier to dental attendance does not necessarily act alone and may combine with such psycho-social factors as dental anxiety and lifestyle. When working together these factors may exacerbate or alleviate time pressures thereby inhibiting or enabling access to dental care, respectively. This situation is illustrated by Case 3.

Case 3

Lack of time was given as a reason for non-attendance by a woman lawyer. She had fractured a molar and a temporary dressing had been placed in the tooth. After a considerable length of time and a number of broken appointments she attended. She admitted that her busy lifestyle was an excuse for broken appointments, 'I find the whole dental business a bit anxiety-provoking' she said 'If I'm honest, it's the local anaesthetic injection that really puts me off'.

In other circumstances dentate status will combine with age and treatment perception[5] to enable or inhibit access to dental attendance. For instance when asked about dental attendance an 80-year-old edentulous woman commented:

> 'I ain't got no teeth so I'm lucky no need to go ... haven't been to the dentist since these teeth were fitted ... that must be ... oh ... at least 20 years ago'.

Whereas a 70-year-old woman with her own teeth perceived dental care as an important part of her overall health care regime:

> 'I'd be worried about what would happen to my teeth if I didn't go ... I don't want too much treatment just enough to make sure my teeth last me out'.

Pre-adolescence and adolescence

Pre-adolescence and adolescence are times when changes are observed in needs perception, dental attendance and compliance with preventive advice. These changes start in pre-adolescence (approximately 12–14 years of age).[14] The pre-adolescent patient who a year or so earlier was so particular about his oral hygiene, now cares little about brushing his teeth. The dentist, when viewing his bite-wings, fears the presence of inter-proximal lesions. Such shifts in compliance with respect to oral hygiene and sugar consumption are to be expected in the pre-adolescent. Associated with this stage of development is a craving for sweet foods and drinks as well as lack of concern for personal hygiene of any kind. The influence of psychological development as a barrier must be recognised by the dental team. Using this information the dental team can gently inform and encourage the pre-adolescent to accept dental care and advice knowing that this is time well spent. Within a short period of time the patient will enter adolescence when a nice smile and appearance become all important.

By the time adolescence[15] is reached psycho-social factors such as parental dental attendance, gender and educational aspirations seem to have positive and negative effects. They may heighten or lower the adolescents' awareness of their dental health needs.[16] For instance, girls and those adolescents intending to enter tertiary education have a more regular pattern of dental attendance compared with boys and those intending to leave school without any qualifications. It would seem that depending on the specific characteristics of the adolescent, dental health care in its widest sense may be disturbed or consolidated during this period of development.

What the dentist is observing in these changing behaviours are the vicissitudes of pre-adolescence and adolescence. During adolescence the psychological changes which occur are due to the adolescents' evolving relationship with their parents. This has consequences for dental attendance and the need to establish a new more adult, real relationship and treatment alliance with the dentist. Therefore on the one hand the dental health professional may be viewed as a parental figure whose authority must be questioned resulting in failed appointments and non-compliance: on the other the adolescents' interest in their appearance[†] may provide the impetus for regular attendance and increased perceptions of treatment need. Understanding the adolescents' seemingly bizarre behaviour will enable the dentist to provide accessible dental health care for this patient group.

Lack of access

While this final barrier may represent more clearly than any other the physical aspects of accessing dental care it also refers to difficulties encountered in relation to problems with communication and language.

Language and communication problems can lead to misunderstandings which exacerbate worries and concerns about dental treatment. In addition to dental fears and costs of dental treatment people from ethnic minority groups, for example, cite language and communication difficulties as considerable barriers to accessing dental care. The dental team which does not appreciate that differences in cultures exist may inadvertently inhibit rather than help their patients access dental care.[17]

With regard to the physical difficulties encountered, lack of access refers to any problem experienced when gaining entrance to practice premises such as wheelchair access to waiting areas, lavatories, the dental surgery itself as well as transport problems and reliance on public transport. Lack of access particularly affects people with special dental health care needs. Older people, those with physical or sensory disabilities and learning difficulties may experience problems when accessing dental care. If this lack of access is due to physical problems experienced at the dental surgery, they will be compounded by the need to use public transport.[4]

Conclusions

It has been proposed that barriers to accessing dental care have their sources within the patient's previous life experiences and their psychosocial background. These factors combine together to construct barriers reducing the patient's ability to access dental health care.

For adult patients the barriers include dental anxiety, financial costs of dental treatment, perceptions of dental need and lack of access. For younger children their barriers to dental care will be affected by parental

---

[†]Health actions which are carried out to improve health are called 'health-directed behaviours'. Those health actions which are carried out to improve appearance (e.g. oral hygiene to have nice smile) and have a health spin off (e.g. less plaque, less gingivitis) are called 'health-related behaviours'. Health-related behaviours provided an important preventive strategy for adolescents.

attitude and anxieties. For pre-adolescents and adolescents dental attendance and compliance with preventive advice will be influenced by their
stage of psychological development. Irrespective of the category of barrier
to accessing dental care it is the place of the dental health professional to
acknowledge that barriers exist and within the two-person endeavour
which is the dentist–patient interaction, assist their patients to access and
accept dental health care.

References

1 Nuttall N. Review of attendance behaviour. *Dent Update* 1997; **24**: 111–113
2 Cohen L K. Converting unmet need for care to effective demand. *Int Dent J* 1987; **37**: 114–116.
3 Finch H, Keegan J, Ward K. *Barriers to the receipt of dental care — a qualitative research study.* London: Social and Community Planning Research, 1988.
4 Adams E K, Freeman R, Gelbier S, Gibson B J. Accessing primary dental care in three inner city boroughs. *Community Dent Health* 1997; **14**: 108–112.
5 Vassend O. Anxiety, pain and discomfort associated with dental treatment *Behav Res Ther* 1993; **31**: 659–666.
6 Liddell A, DiFazio L, Blackwood J, Ackerman C. Long-term follow-up of treated dental phobics. *Behav Res Ther* 1994; **32**: 605–610.
7 Corah N L. Development of a dental anxiety scale. *J Dent Res* 1969; 48: 596.
8 Humphris G M, Morrison T, Lindsay S J. The Modified Dental Anxiety Scale: validation and United Kingdom norms. *Community Dent Health* 1995; **12**: 143–150.
9 Venham L L, Gaulin-Kremer E. A self-report measure of situational anxiety for young children. *Pediatr Dent.* 1979; **1**:91–96.
10 Carson P, Freeman R. Assessing child dental anxiety: the validity of clinical observations. *Int J Pediatr Dent* 1997; **7**: 171–176
11 Carson P, Freeman R. Tell–show–do: reducing anticipatory anxiety in emergency paediatric dental patients. *Int J Health Prom Edu* 1998; **36**: 87–90.
12 Call R L. The effects of poverty on children's dental health. *Pediatrician* 1989; **16**: 200–206.
13 Gibson B J, Drennan J, Hanna S, Freeman R. Routine dentaling and the six monthly check-up. *J Dent Res* 1997; **76**: 1046
14 Freud A.(1949) On certain difficulties in the preadolescent's relation to his parents. In *The Selected Anna Freud* (Eds. R Ekins, R Freeman) Harmondsworth: Penguin Books, 1998.
15 Freud A.(1958) Adolescence. In *The Selected Anna Freud* (Eds. R Ekins, R Freeman) Harmondsworth: Penguin, 1998.
16 Freeman R, Maizels J, Wyllie M, Sheiham A. The relationship between health related knowledge, attitudes and dental health behaviours in 14–16 year old adolescents. *Community Dent Health* 1993; **10**: 397–403.
17 Williams S A, Gelbier S. Dentists and ethnic minority communities. *Br Dent J* 1989; **166**: 194–195.

Barriers to accessing dental care: dental health professional factors

Cohen[1] in her report on the FDI's classification of barriers to dental attendance stated that factors associated with the dental health professional had to be considered if dentist are to provide accessible dental health care for patients. The FDI stated that barriers in relation to the dental profession included:

> ...*inappropriate manpower resources, uneven geographical distribution, training inappropriate to changing needs and demands and insufficient sensitivity to patient's attitudes and needs.*

If this category of barriers is to be applied to those working in general practice then they must be considered within the same category headings as for the patient (see Chapter 6). For instance 'inappropriate manpower resources' and 'uneven geographical distribution' are commensurate with the patient category 'lack of access', 'training inappropriate to changing needs and demands' is equivalent to 'perception of needs', while 'insufficient sensitivity to patient's attitudes and needs', could be thought of as the influence of psycho-social factors such as occupational stress, time urgency and financial considerations with regard to the viability of the practice.

Ms A's responses to John (Case 1) provide an opportunity to examine how the FDI's classification of dental profession barriers can be applied to the general practice setting. There can be little doubt that Ms A in her relationship with John exhibits two if not three of the barriers to which Cohen[1] refers. The barriers constructed by Ms A could also be thought of as psychosocial influences with occupational stress, financial considerations, perceptions of John's needs and time urgency playing a role in Ms A's responses to provide accessible dental care for her pre-adolescent patient.

Case 1

John is 12 years old and has an uneasy working relationship with his dentist, Ms A. She, on her part, responds badly to this anxious pre-adolescent, feeling that treating him is a waste of time and effort. She hates to see John's name in the appointment book and even at the prospect of treating him becomes irritable. John has, to quote Ms A, 'got under my skin'. She admitted that she has even thought that she could avoid treating him by being on leave when his next routine examination was due.

Thinking in this way permits an alternative view of barriers as a consequence of the dentist–patient interaction. It is proposed that since equivalent barriers exist for both patient and dentist, it is their interaction which reduces the dentist's ability to furnish accessible dental care and the patient's ability to access the service provided. It is the interaction and combination of dentist barriers with those of the patient that makes dental care inaccessible. If dentists are to assist people access routine care then they must be aware of their own role in limiting access and compliance.

Psycho-social factors

Occupational stress

The idea that dentistry is the most stressful of all of the health professions was first proposed by Cooper et al[2,3]. In the 1980s Cooper et al[2,3] proposed that occupational stress was due to:

> ...time-related pressures, fearful patients, high case loads, financial worries, problems with staff, equipment breakdowns, defective materials, poor working conditions and the routine and boring nature of the job.

By the 1990s Humphris and Cooper[4] had identified four, new, additional stressors. These included concerns about the future of general practice dentistry, aggressive and hostile patients, worries about the risk of cross infection and fears about litigation. There could be little doubt that the dental profession was being repeatedly exposed to a variety of sources of occupational stress. For some the effects of occupational stress would be minimal and would be confined to feelings of concern about practice policy or worries about a particular patient. The case of Ms A and John is illustrative in this regard. For others occupational stress would have detrimental effects in that not only could these susceptible individuals suffer physical and/or emotional ill health (emotional exhaustion) but they could also experience a withdrawal of interest from their work (lowered personal achievement) and a turning away from patients and colleagues alike (depersonalisation).[5] A dental health professional who found herself in this position was said to be suffering from 'burn-out'.[6]

The 'burnt-out dentist'

Stress and anxieties together with a withdrawal of interest from work inhibit dental health professionals from providing accessible dental care for their patients.[6] The 'burnt-out' dentist who encounters a dentally anxious patient will be unable to deal or help the patient cope with her dental fears. The patient's dental anxiety in combination with the dentist's own occupational stress allows a situation to occur in which barriers to providing or accepting dental care result. An example of this is the case of Mr O (Case 2). His withdrawal of interest, together with his anxiety resulted in his impatience with a dentally anxious emergency patient. Mr O was unable to cope with his own stresses and his patient's anxieties which resulted in the patient deciding to access care elsewhere.

Case 2

Mr O's dental nurse had noticed a change in his manner and demeanour in the last few months. Mr O had become withdrawn and had lost interest in his work. He couldn't even bring himself to speak to his patients. In the previous week a dentally anxious patient who arrived as an emergency was the last straw. He didn't have time for her. On previous occasions Mr O would have discussed the proposed treatment with the patient. This time he told the patient the tooth needed to be extracted and did it. The patient confided to the receptionist that she had been told that Mr O was good with nervous patients. She had thought of registering in the practice but he seemed so disinterested there didn't seem much point in becoming a patient here.

The importance of recognising that dental health professionals are constantly being bombarded by stressors allows them to appreciate the potential for 'burn-out'. Dentists who can structure their time effectively and can acknowledge their difficulties with patients and staff members are in a better position to cope with occupational stress. It is their awareness and ability to acknowledge the existence of stressors in the workplace which allows them to cope effectively with stress, prevent 'burn-out' and maintain an accessible dental service for their patients.

Financial costs

Issues associated with the running costs of a viable dental practice have been highlighted as problem areas with respect to maintaining an accessible general dental practice. Concerns and worries about how the financial viability of a practice would be affected by providing specific forms of dental care for specific patient groups has been shown to reduce practice accessibility.

The relationship between obtaining the target income and providing an accessible dental practice has been shown to influence practice policy with regard to special needs patients. Dentists in general dental practice, while providing dental care for patients with special dental needs, only do so for those who can access the care they provide.[6] Hence there remains a group of patients who are unable to access care in the usual manner. Dentists and/or practice managers have stated that their concerns about the financial burden to the practice prohibit them from providing accessible care for this sub-group of special needs patients.[7–9] Links between running costs, time urgency and stress were highlighted as factors prohibiting the provision of dental care for patients with special dental needs. With regard to providing specific forms of dental treatment, such as relative analgesia or domicillary dental care, they again pointed to their concerns about the financial implications[10] this would have for their practices.

Viability of the practice

The perception that providing, for example, a domicillary dental service would be detrimental to the viability of the practice was questioned by dentists who had not had previous or current experience of this type of service provision. A general practitioner who ran a domicillary dental service for many years and was able to provide a range of restorative, prosthetic and periodontal treatments for his house-bound patients, questioned his colleagues' concerns. He remembered his worries about providing this type of service and how it would disturb his practice but his concerns proved unrealistic. He had managed to organise his schedule to allow the service to become an integral part of his practice profile.

He acknowledged, 'Until you have had personal experience of this type of service you think I must be mad and I'll go bankrupt but it's not like that, you just organise the visits when time's available, you work in the appointments and incorporate them into your clinical routines'.

Nevertheless time urgency and worries about income can promote barriers in some busy general practices. This was the case for Mr X and Sally. Sally, aged 12 years, was frightened of the drill and local anaesthetic injection. Mr X had tried on several occasions to persuade Sally to accept local anaesthetic with attempts to use relative analgesia also failing. Mr X decided to refer Sally for restorative treatment under general anaesthetic. His reasons were quite clear:

'First, it was doing the child no good ... then it was doing me no good, I started to feel irritated with her. I was wasting a lot of my time and her mother's. I kept thinking, when I was trying to give her the local, of the other patients in the waiting room and I thought I can't afford this.'

Perceptions of need

Perceptions of dental need are based upon the clinical training of dental health professionals. The normative need[11] (see Chapter 2) provides the basis from which treatment plans are formulated, negotiated and discussed with patients. A consequence of the identification of a clinical treatment need is that it facilitates access to secondary level care. The reason for the dentist's course of action may be related to concerns about embarking on a course of treatment. In this way the dentist is in fact reducing the patient's access to primary dental care. The decision to refer the patient with severe periodontal disease for specialist care[12] or a small child with an acute abscess to a centre of excellence for a general anaesthetic extraction, is consistent with the normative need. In either clinical situation the decision to refer may reduce access to the practice but facilitate patient entry to secondary level care.

Another clinical situation exists, however, when the dental health professional's perception of the patient's needs are not in harmony with the patient. An example of this dichotomy may be the patient's wish for anterior restorations prior to posterior ones and the dentist's plan to complete the posterior amalgams prior to the anterior restorations. Such clinical situations as this, can be managed, with the dentist and patient arriving at an accommodation. However, when the patient insists that treatment is needed which is thought to be contra-indicated, difficulties in patient management start to emerge.

A perfect dentition

An example of this is the yearning for a perfect dentition.[13] The majority of patients who present for cosmetic dentistry are satisfied and pleased with the outcome of their treatment, but occasionally a patient presents who on completion of treatment is distraught and demands that the veneers be removed or the crowns replaced. The intensity and the inappropriateness of their reaction to dental care, their insistence that the crowns look ugly and ridiculous, their intense anxiety accompanied by a refusal to leave their homes suggests that all is not well. In this scenario the dentist is in the middle of a clinical dilemma. On the one hand he can see little clinically wrong with the crowns but on the other he is faced with a dissatisfied patient.

In the examples that follow the first practitioner was at a loss since she could see little wrong with the veneers she had fitted but nevertheless at the patient's insistence she removed them. In the second example the patient's odd behaviour during two preliminary consultations raised the practitioner's concerns with regard to the treatment outcome. In both situations it was the mismatch in need perception which resulted in a clinical dilemma that affected the provision of dental health care. The need for careful and sensitive questioning (see Chapter 8) when assessing patients demanding cosmetic dentistry, may be necessary in order to prevent difficult encounters in clinical practice.

While mismatches in perception of need may cause barriers to be erected, sometimes the dentist's responses to the normative need together with the patients' wishes for dental care are appropriate. Acknowledging

Case 3

A married woman aged 40 years old had porcelain veneers placed upon her upper and lower central incisors to reduce upper and lower mid-line diastemae. The patient's appearance was greatly improved and the treatment was considered a success by all involved. When the patient returned several days later in an acutely anxious and distressed state the dentist was understandably confused as to the patient's extreme reaction. The patient insisted that the veneers were removed and, in order to help the patient, the dentist complied with her wishes. However even now several years later, the patient still feels that her teeth are deformed and that if only she could have her teeth perfect she would be free of her anxieties and difficulties.

Case 4

A married man aged 30 presented requesting veneers. On examination he had tetracycline staining which although noticeable was not disfiguring. During the history taking the patient's wife insisted that her husband had wanted veneers for at least the last 10 years. The patient remained silent. A second consultation prior to the start of treatment was suggested by the dentist. During this second meeting the patient remained silent except for an outburst when he insisted that he had always wanted perfect teeth. He felt that veneers would be the solution to his problem. His withdrawn state and anxiety during the two consultations together with his inappropriate outburst caused the dentist to have great concerns about embarking upon treatment. In particular the dentist feared the patient's response and satisfaction with the outcome of the proposed cosmetic treatment.

the appropriateness and inappropriateness of their responses in relation to patients' wishes will allow dental health professionals to provide accessible dental health care.

Lack of access

Lack of access as a psycho-social factor in maintaining an accessible dental practice relates not only to the physical characteristics of the practice premises (ramps, lifts, wide corridors, etc.) but also to the provision of care for dentally anxious patients (psychological accessibility) as well as having the appropriate auxiliary personnel.[7]

The physical accessibility of a practice has been shown to be associated with the demographic profile of the practice principal. The fewer the years in practice, the more postgraduate courses attended, the decision to provide weekend emergency dental care are all important characteristics in maintaining a practice with high physical accessibility.[7]

A similar demographic profile has been demonstrated by practitioners who provide relative analgesia services[7,10] in their practices and in this way allow for the treatment of patients with psychological special needs. Psychological accessibility also relates to the dental health professional's ability to communicate effectively with patients. This ability has been shown to be greater in younger, more recently qualified dentists and in women dental health professionals. These practitioners tended to listen more to their patients and attempt to provide care in keeping with the expressed needs of their adult and child patients.[7,10]

The dental team working together will also be able to increase accessibility for dental health care. In this regard the receptionist, the dental nurse and hygienist are invaluable. The receptionist can increase accessibility by judicious use of the appointment book. The dental nurse can increase accessibility, not only by her patient management but also in her surgery work with the dentist.[14] The hygienist working with her dental colleagues enables more patients to access preventive health care by providing the practice with her expert oral health promotion.

The demographic and patient management skills of the dental health professional are not the only characteristics which should be considered in relation to lack of access. Other salient features which should be included are surgery hours and position and location of the dental practice. It has been shown that patients use health services which are within a 6 mile (10 kilometre) radius of their homes, work or schools.[15] The relation between access, location and distance travelled has been identified by industry with many of the larger multinationals providing in-house dental care facilities — thus improving access to care. Similarly the community dental service has provided mobile dental units for school children and patients with special needs. As practice position and location are known to increase accessibility the majority of surgeries are positioned on main bus routes and located in the shopping areas. This has been developed further with a pharmaceutical company intending to provide dental health care facilities in retail locations.

Conclusions

It has been proposed that barriers to accessing dental health care exist not only in relation to the patient but also in relation to the dentist together with the characteristics of the practice. It has been suggested that within the two-person endeavour which is the dentist–patient interaction that equivalent concerns and anxieties are experienced by both dentist and patient. It has been postulated that it is this mirroring of concerns — occupational stress and dental anxiety for dentist and patient respectively — which provides the ingredients for a barrier to be erected that reduces access to regular dental care. Dentists, by being aware of the potential for the construction of barriers can, by developing their patient management skills and changing practice policy, maintain and provide an accessible dental health care service for their patients.

References

1 Cohen L K. Converting unmet need for care to effective demand. *Int Dent J* 1987; **37**: 114-116.
2 Cooper C L, Mallinger M, Kahn R. Identifying sources of occupational stress in dentists. *J Occupational Psych* 1981; **51**: 227-234.
3 Cooper C L, Watts J, Kelly M. Job satisfaction, mental health and job stressors among general dental practitioners. *Brit Dent J* 1987; **162**: 77-81.
4 Humphris G M, Cooper C L. New stressors for general dental practitioners in the past 10 years: a qualitative study. *Brit Dent J* 1998; **185**: 404-406
5 Maslach C, Goldberg J. Prevention of burnout: new perspectives. *App and Prevent Psych* 1998; **7**: 63-74
6 Burke F J T, Main J R, Freeman R. The practice of dentistry: a review of occupational stress and assessment of reasons for premature retirement. *Br Dent J* 1997; **182**: 250-254.
7 Freeman R, Adams E K, Gelbier S. The provision of primary dental care for patients with special needs. *Primary Dent Care* 1997; **4**: 31-34.
8 Freeman R, Adams E K. The prediction of dentists' work behaviour; factors affecting choice or intention in the treatment of special need patients. *Community Dent Health*. 1991; **8**: 213-219
9 Gibson B J, Freeman R. Dangerousness and dentistry: an explanation of dentists' reactions and responses to the treatment of HIV-Seropositive patients. *Community Dent and Oral Epidemol* 1996; **24**: 341-345.
10 Carson P. *Paediatric sedation and general anaesthetic services: choices for the future.* Belfast: The Queen's University of Belfast, 1998. Unpublished PhD thesis.
11 Ong B N. *The practice of health services research.* London: Chapman & Hall, 1993.
12 Freeman R, Linden G L. Health directed and health related dimensions of oral health behaviours of periodontal referrals. *Community Dent Health* 1995; **12**: 48-51.
13 Freeman R, Kells B. A dysmorphophobic reaction to cosmetic dentistry: observations and responses to psychotherapeutic intervention. *Psychoanalytic Psychotherapy* 1996; **10**: 21-31.
14 Gibson B J, Freeman R, Ekins R. The role of the dental nurse in general practice: introducing the concept of dental housewifeing. *Br Dent J* 1999; **186**: 213-215.
15 Jacob C, Plamping D. *The practice of primary health care.* Bristol: Wright, 1989.

Communicating effectively: some practical suggestions

The first steps in understanding responses and reactions to dental health care is to glean information about the patients. Dental health professionals must try to know about their patients' psychosocial background as well as gaining an understanding of their own reactions to the care they provide. Recognising patient and professional factors which singly or in combination affect surgery routines allows the influence of psychological and social factors to be contained. Reducing barriers and resistances, in this way, strengthens the treatment alliance (see Chapter 1), thereby enabling patients to accept and comply with preventive dental health care advice and restorative treatment plans, being offered and provided.[1,2]

If dental health professionals are to provide holistic health care and promote self-reliance in their patients, they must know their patients. They do this by considering important episodes in their patients' lives, by knowing problems or difficulties their patients encounter and by recognising their patients apprehensiveness about dental treatment. All available means to access patient information must be used. Dental health professionals must be proficient in their communication skills. For instance, the setting for the interview with patients must be empathetic.[3–5] They must encourage their patients to ventilate their feelings, thoughts, worries and fears in relation to treatment and its outcome, as well as ensuring that their patients fully understand what is being said. The health professionals, the dentist, hygienist and dental nurse, must accept that their patients' feelings about dental health care may be at odds with their own and, as such, may stir strong counter-feelings or reactions. These feelings must be understood so that agreed treatment may proceed.[6,7] Dental health practitioners must walk the tightrope between being objective on the one hand, and empathetic on the other, with regard to their patients' needs. The ability to achieve a balance between objectivity and empathy is the essence of effective communication.[3-5]

There can be little doubt that this is a tall order. The dentist, hygienist, and dental nurse within their busy work schedule have little if any time for prolonged patient interviews. Somehow they must find a system which permits the elicitation of patient details in as short a time as possible. Effective communication provides the dental health professional with a strategy by which this may be achieved.[5,6] All the information needed to care for, and to negotiate preventive and treatment plans with patients may be obtained using the effective communication strategy entitled 'CLASS'.[8] 'CLASS' provides and enables dental health practitioners to become proficient in their information retrieval. The acronym 'CLASS' stands for:

1. C   the physical Context of the clinical encounter
         — the empathetic setting
2. L   the Listening and questioning skills of the dental
         health professional
3. A   practitioners' Acknowledgement of their feelings
         and those of the patient
4. S   the development of a preventive and restorative
         treatment Strategy negotiated with the patient
         (see Chapter 9)
5. S   providing a Summary of treatment and preventive
         options (Figure 8.1).[8]

The application and suitability of 'CLASS' for dental health care can be revealed by showing how they inter-connect with the key aspects or elements of effective communication. In the first communication elements (see above) the 'C' (for the physical setting of the interview), 'L' (for listening skills), 'A' (for acknowledging feelings) and 'S' (for negotiating treatment plans) from the strategy are evident. In the communication elements 4 and 5, the 'L' (for listening skills), 'A' (for acknowledging feelings), together with the two final 'Ss' (for providing summaries and feedback) may be clearly shown (Figure 8.1). The clinical application of the final 'Ss' are also relevant for the motivation of patients as detailed in Chapter 9.

The key elements of effective communication[9,10]

Communication is a two-way process in which verbal utterances and non-verbal cues are used within the dentist-patient interaction. Sometimes during these exchanges it may seem as if the practitioner is doing nothing, just listening, (passive). The patient appears to be doing everything (active) by talking and describing symptoms or how they feel about treatment. This is a difficult situation for dentists because usually it is the dentist who is active and the patient who is passive — an apparent reversal of roles.

To think of communication as individuals talking at each other, would be to ignore the essence of effective communication.[5] The importance of knowing the patient's symptoms, feelings and psycho-social background makes information retrieval a most active aspect of patient care. When the dentist appears to be passive (s)he is in fact being active, by watching the patients' behaviour (non-verbal cues) and listening, thus encouraging the patient to speak freely (verbal communication).

Non-verbal communications

It has been said that 65% of all communication is non-verbal.[11] Non-verbal communications or cues are more readily believed than those of the spoken word. It is the case, for people in general, that 'actions speak louder than words'.

The first element of communication is an understanding of the patient's non-verbal communication.[12] This includes not only the context of the interview, but also, the level and position of the patient, proximity, how close the practitioner is to the patient (the invasion of a the personal space), the patient's posture (how they are lying in the dental chair), eye contact between the dentist and patient as well as the non-verbal reinforcers of speech — that is the 'ahs', 'ers' and 'uhms'. In this regard non-verbal communication reflects clearly the 'C' of the 'CLASS' communication strategy (Figure 8.1).[8]

A way of putting patients at ease and hence engaging and facilitating conversation is to make eye contact with the patient. Case 1 illustrates when eye contact is absent.

Case 1

Sheena, a 10-year-old girl, had arrived for impression for a gum shield. She was learning to play hockey. Mother and Sheena were brought into the surgery. The dentist, who was running late, gruffly asked Mother and Sheena to be seated. Impression trays were chosen. As the impression material was being mixed Sheena wriggled in the chair. Mother got up to comfort her daughter holding her hand tightly while the impressions were recorded. Sheena's worries went unnoticed by the dentist who had paid little if any attention to her. Mother later commented upon her own discomfort during the appointment.

The C-L-A-S-S Communication Strategy[8]		
Acronym	Meaning	Skills needed
C	The Context of the interview	providing an empathetic setting, maintaining eye contact, knowledge of body language
L	Listening skills	helping people to talk, using open questions, active listening
A	Acknowledging feelings	acknowledging feelings, empathy, clarifying, reflecting, paraphrasing using people's own words
S	Strategy	assessing patient's treatment expectations, developing, proposing and negotiating treatment and preventive plans
S	Summary	providing a summary of treatment and preventive option, obtaining feedback

**Figure 8.1
The class
communication
strategy**

Listening

Listening skills are perhaps the most important of all of the verbal communication skills.[10] Often listening is felt to have a passive quality. However, listening is one of the most active elements of verbal communication. The aim of active listening is to engage, facilitate and encourage the patient to speak.[13] This aspect of listening is reflected in the skills needed in the 'L' part of the 'CLASS' strategy.[8]

Listening is not simply hearing words. It involves a concerted effort to listen to the way the words are said, to recognise the feelings underlying the spoken word and to be aware of what the patient has left out of their narrative. This last aspect of listening has been called 'listening with the third ear'.[6] Often what is left out or unsaid provides the practitioner with important material concerning the patients' resistances to accepting dental treatment (see Chapter 5). Case 2 is illustrative of how treatment needs can go unnoticed when patients leave things unsaid. In this example the patient's

Case 2

A woman dentist had completed treatment for an elderly house-bound patient. The patient enjoyed seeing the young dentist who was always courteous and cheerful. The complete dentures were duly inserted and the dentist agreed a time with the patient to check the new dentures. At the next visit the patient assured the dentist that the dentures were perfect. In fact the patient had told the home help that the dentures looked lovely but he 'couldn't wear them when eating — they rubbed'. He had not mentioned anything to the dentist 'cause [he] hadn't wanted to upset her'.

reticence in telling the dentist how uncomfortable he found wearing his new dentures was associated with his liking for the dentist and his concerns that she would be angry if he were critical of 'the teeth'.

In Case 3 the dentist, Mr T, did listen to what had been left out by Emma's mother. He was aware of the difficulties Emma's mother had in saying how cross she had been with him at a previous appointment for not being available for her daughter. By acknowledging the anger of Emma's mother Mr T was able to restore contact.

Case 3

Mother returned after many months with her daughter Emma, aged 7. Emma was now in pain which served to increase Emma's anxieties about treatment. Mr T was most concerned and asked why they had waited so long before coming to see him. Mother was silent. Mr T, now remembered, that he had been ill and Emma had been treated by a colleague. When he broached this with mother, she was able to say that Emma had been very upset not to see Mr T. At the last appointment they had been kept waiting, then they had been told that Mr T was not available. It seemed to mother that Emma was 'being passed from pillar to post ... no-one was interested in [her] daughter's dental health'.

If dentists are to provide dental health care for their patients then they must encourage their patients to speak freely. They do this by active listening. Active listening will be achieved by conducting the interview in a non-threatening and empathetic setting. Dental health professionals must give attention to what is being said and be able to reflect, clarify and paraphrase the patients' words. Finally they must ensure that they have understood the patients' message conveyed in their conversation with them.

Engaging the patient (Figure 8.2)
Engaging
Engaging the patient in conversation may be split into 3 phases which are reflected in the 'C', 'L', 'A' and 'S' of the 'CLASS' strategy.[8] The first phase is associated with encouraging the patient to talk freely and without difficulty. The second phase is associated with explaining or making sure patients understand what has been discussed and is characterised by negotiating treatment and preventive plans. The third and final phase, is associated with clarifying the patients' expressed and felt needs, with regard to treatment plans and outcome expectations. For each phase of the interview the dental health professional uses specific questioning which enables the patients to describe the history of their presenting complaint, divulge their medical histories, talk about their previous dental experiences and clarify negotiated treatment plans.

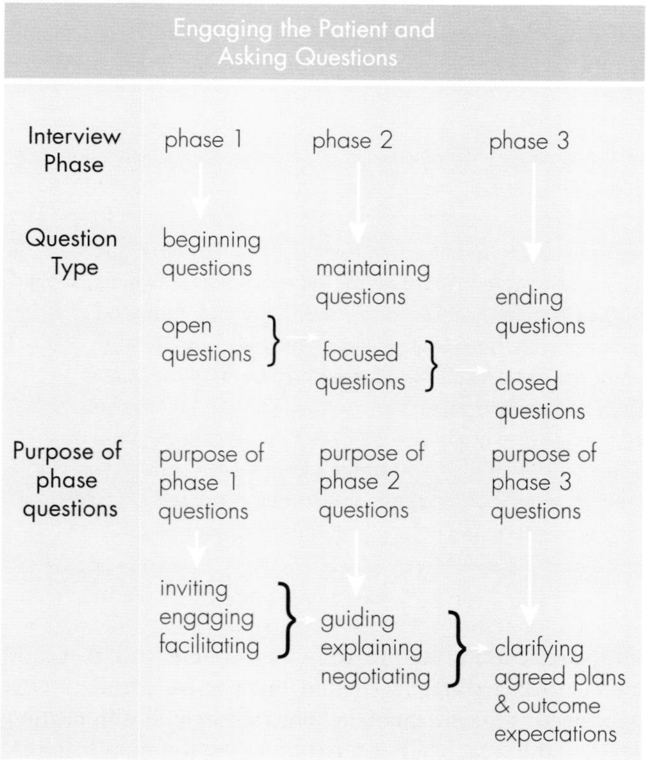

Figure 8.2 Engaging the patient and asking questions

Phase 1: beginning or open questions[9,10] During phase 1, beginning or open questions are used to invite and engage the patient in conversation. This allows the patient to talk and to bring as much or as little information they feel is necessary, or wish to impart, during the interview. By allowing the patient to set the agenda, in this way, open questions facilitate information gathering.

Phase 2: maintaining or focused questions[9,10] In phase 2 of the interview focused questions are used to forge and maintain the impetus of the interview. It is during this phase of the conversation that the dental health professional may need to explain treatment plans and ensure that the patient has understood what has been suggested, or the dental health education advice which has been given. Focused questions often say 'I appreciate that it is hard to tell me about it (guidance) but you must try (support). Focused questions of this second type provide support for the patient when talking about difficult issues by guiding them through the interview.

In Case 4, focused questions of a supporting format were used to help Mrs A speak of a personal tragedy which occurred prior to the onset of her burning mouth syndrome.

Case 4

Mrs A, aged 45 years old, had been referred to a specialist clinic with burning mouth syndrome of three months duration. She was low spirited, tearful and had no interest in her appearance (*non-verbal cues*). She was asked: 'What happened before the burning started ?' (*focused question*). With great difficulty Mrs A stated that her only daughter had been killed in a car accident 15 months previously. This had been a shock from which she would never recover but she hoped 'she'd come to terms with it'. It occurred to her as she spoke that the burning started 3 months ago on the anniversary of her daughter's death.'

Explaining

Explaining is a fundamental aspect and an integral part of negotiating treatment options and health goals with patients. Explanations and dental health advice must be clear, concise and to the point. In this way the amount of dental health education given must be restricted to 3 or 4 essential points. These must be expressed in ordinary language, given early in the interview and repeated several times. It is during this time that the dental health professional must ensure that the patient has understood the information.[14] In the following illustration although the dentist thought she had explained the results of the biopsy it was apparent that she had not ensured the patient had understood what she had said and the patient had remained confused about the outcome of the surgical procedure.

Case 5

Mr N, a 60-year-old man, returned for the results of a biopsy of a lesion from the lateral border of his tongue. The history and clinical examination suggested a diagnosis of a squamous cell papilloma. A biopsy was performed to confirm this. The dentist told Mr N that 'growth on the side of the tongue was a little wart'. Mr N nodded. The consultation ended. On his way out Mr N asked if the results of the test were OK. The dentist realised that Mr N had not understood. She explained that he had nothing to worry about. He had a little wart in his mouth like children sometimes have on their hands.

Guiding, supporting and negotiating
Focused questions, which guide and support the patient to express uncomfortable or difficult thoughts about personal difficulties or the care they have received, are useful when the dental health professional wishes to deal quickly with a patient's concerns. This form of question indicates to the patients that the dentist has acknowledged the difficulty they are experiencing and will support them in expressing their thoughts. This was the situation with Mrs Q who felt that she was being fobbed off despite feeling her teeth were sensitive after completion of her dental treatment.

Phase 3: ending or closed questions.[9,10] Closed questions are important as they clarify important points brought to the interview by the patient. They are in essence yes/no questions and are often used towards the end of the interview. For instance, in the case of Mrs Q they were used to clarify that she had agreed treatment with the practice hygienist. At other times they will be used to clarify the patients' expectations of treatment.

Leading questions[9]
Finally a word of caution with regard to questioning. Leading questions such as, 'You haven't had rheumatic fever have you?' are to be avoided. Some patients will agree with the questioner although they may not understand the content of the question.

Case 6

Mrs Q, a 55-year-old woman, requested an appointment with her dentist. She had had a number of fillings replaced and was dissatisfied with them. She complained bitterly that her teeth felt sharp and were sensitive. She had had none of these symptoms before. She stated that: 'One must never be critical of professional people be they doctors, lawyers or even dentists'. Her dentist commented that the last thing she would like to be was critical of him (focused question). This enabled Mrs Q to state that she would not wish to be critical but she was cross at the way she felt he had treated her teeth. This allowed the dentist to explain and show Mrs Q again that the sensitivity she experienced was due to 'receding gums'. The dentist gently suggested (negotiating) that an appointment with the practice hygienist would be a good idea. Mrs Q gratefully accepted this treatment suggestion.

Acknowledging thoughts and feelings

In the 'CLASS'[8] acronym A stands for acknowledging the patients' and practitioners' feelings, attitudes and thoughts. In this section rather than concentrating upon the patient, the thoughts, experiences and feelings of the dental health professional will be examined.[6,7,12,15] The reason for doing this is to appreciate how the practitioner's counter-reactions may distort the communication process. When communication breakdown occurs barriers may be set up which may inhibit patients accessing and accepting dental health care.

Three vignettes are relevant in this regard. They illustrate how the practitioner's counter-reactions to the patient's responses to treatment may result in communication breakdown and patient loss. In Case 7, the patient's continuous complaints engendered a sense of gloom in the staff of a pain clinic who dreaded his monthly appointments. In Case 8, the dentist was shocked

Case 7

Mr X complained bitterly about his painful teeth. At times he felt he wanted them all taken out and he would wear dentures. His continual complaints resulted in a sense of despondency and hopelessness in the dental staff who cared for him at the specialist pain clinic. They felt they could do little to help and listened in silence to his complaints and grumbles.

by the patient's distress at the extraction of her remaining teeth. Although this patient was lost to the practice, the practice regime was changed with each patient being counselled prior to the extraction of their anterior teeth. Case 9 shows how awareness of counter-reactions promotes self-esteem in the dental health professional and her patients.

Case 8

Mrs D agreed to have her remaining teeth extracted and an immediate complete upper denture inserted at the extraction visit. The extractions were performed. Suddenly Mrs D cried inconsolably stating that she had not realised how important her remaining few teeth had been to her. Her distress shocked the dentist who later admitted how guilty she felt about the extractions and the denture. In consultation with practice colleagues it was agreed that future patients would be 'counselled' prior to the extraction of any upper anterior teeth.

Case 9

Ms B, the practice hygienist had been asked to see Mr E again to give him advice about his tooth brushing and oral hygiene. The thought of seeing this patient, yet again, filled Ms B with despondency — nothing it seemed could be done for him. Being aware of her gloomy feelings, Ms B decided that she would try a new tactic. She organised to video Mr E brushing his teeth. They watched the video together. It was apparent to both Ms B and Mr E that he had not understood what he had been advised to do. Armed with this knowledge a new preventive plan was devised and negotiated. This resulted in great improvements in Mr E's oral hygiene.

Summarising and giving feedback

As the interview nears its close the dental health professional must ensure that the patient has understood what has been discussed. The dentist must summarise (as denoted by the 'S' in the 'CLASS' strategy[8]) the information for the patient. The practitioner knows the patient, and can summarise the necessary clinical or health education information in a manner and in language the patient can understand. By making use of non-verbal communication[12] the dentist can be confident that the patient is agreeable to the negotiated way forward and has grasped the implications with regard to treatment outcome.[10,14]

Giving feedback may be used as a means of bringing the conversation or clinical session to a close. It is at this time that patients may be congratulated upon coping with their dental fears during treatment or upon their improved tooth brushing technique. Feedback allows the dentist to forge and strengthen the treatment alliance (see Chapter 1), thereby empowering and promoting self-reliance in their patients.

Conclusions

This chapter has attempted to set out an effective communication strategy based upon the acronym 'CLASS'. This communication framework has been used widely within medicine and has been useful in helping patients accept health care advice, negotiate treatment proposals and realise the implications of their treatment decisions.

It is applicable for dentistry as it provides the means by which dental health professionals can get to know their patients and ensure that they understand what has been said to them. By being proficient in effective communication dentists and their team can assist and motivate their patients to better oral health.

References

1 Ong L M L, De Haes J C J M, Hoos A M, Lammes F B. Doctor–patient communication: a review of the literature. *Social Science and Medicine* 1995; **40**: 903-918.
2 Sondell K, Soderfeldt B. Dentist-patient communication: a review of relevant models. *Acta Odontol Scand* 1997; **55**: 116-126.
3 Suchman A L, Markakis K, Beckman H B, Frankel R. A model of empathetic communication in the medical interview. *JAMA* 1997; **277**: 678-682.
4 Ptacek J T, Eberhardt T L. Breaking bad news. A review of the literature. *JAMA* 1996; **276**: 296-502.
5 Hirschman S M, Hittleman E. Effective communication. *Gen Dent* 1978; **26**: 38-46.
6 Freeman R. Communication, body language and dental anxiety. *Dent Update* 1992; **19**: 307-309.
7 Freeman R. Using continuous heart rate monitoring to investigate anxiety and its communication within the dentist-patient interaction. *Psychology and Health* 1989; **3**: 307-318.
8 Buckman R, Korsch B, Baile W. *A practical guide to communication skills in clinical practice.* New York: Medical Audio Visual Communications Inc, 1998.
9 Jacob C, Plamping D. *The Practice of Primary Health Care.* Bristol: Wright, 1989.
10 Fielding R. *Clinical communication skills.* Hong Kong: Hong Kong University Press, 1995
11 Argyle M. *Social Interaction.* London: Methuen, 1973.
12 Waitzkin H. Doctor–patient communication: clinical implications of social-scientific research. *JAMA* 1984; **252**: 2441-2446.
13 Kacperek L. Non-verbal communication: the importance of listening *Br J Nurs* 1997; **6**: 275-279.
14 Calkins D R, Davis R B, Reiley P, Phillips R S, Pineo K L C, Delbanco L, Iezzoni L I. Patient–physician communication at hospital discharge and patients' understanding of the postdischarge treatment plan. *Arch Intern Med* 1997; **157**: 1026-1030.
15 Bernzweig J, Takayama J I, Phibbs C, Lewis C, Pantell R H. Gender differences in physician–patient communication: evidence from paediatric visits. *Arch Pediatr Adolesc* 1997; **151**: 586-591

Strategies for motivating the non-compliant patient

The word motivation is often used by dentists to describe their patients' non-compliance with recommended preventive actions. Colloquially motivation seems to refer to anything from the patients' lack of understanding and apparent inability to listen, to changing their health behaviours. It is as if the patient, like a naughty child, is being purposively irritating and is ignoring the advice being given. However, within this clinical scenario, no allowance is made for whether patients have the listening skills or the wish to change, or whether the clinician can listen, provide appropriate amounts of information and be patient enough to allow new health behaviours to become established. These important aspects of behaviour change are absent in discussions and complaints about disinterested and apparently unmotivated patients. It is the role of the dental health professional to assist patients to attain and maintain their oral health. In order to do so dentists must free themselves from any preconceptions or previous experiences of health education. Thus they can examine new ways to enable their patients to adopt and maintain oral health.

Advice-giving strategies for motivation and compliance

Most health education is given in the form of advice and the advice is usually given in the form of knowledge. It has been assumed that by providing knowledge there will be a modification in attitude which will result in behaviour change. The advice model of health education (KAB)[1] is based upon the idea that by increasing patient's awareness of the severity and threat of the disease (the cons) together with the benefits of complying with the recommended preventive actions (the pros) will result in a lasting behaviour change.[1] Essentially, this model proposes that patients can move from a state of being unaware of the need to change to a state of complete compliance with the recommended actions. However, the advice approach to motivating patients is flawed.[2] The problem with giving advice is that, although there may be some short-term benefits, for the most part the advice is largely ignored. The limitations of the advice strategy include the behavioural aim of the intervention, the methods used, the time given for imparting the information, the inertia of mental life (resistances) and the ambivalence or disinterest on either the dentist's or patient's part.

In general practice dental health professionals use advice to help to persuade their patients to adopt preventive actions. Patients hear the advice as critical and intrusive. The patients' resistance to change is increased and unhealthy behaviours reinstated.[3] Dental health professionals, sensing that their words are ignored, feel that dental health education is a waste of time. Brief advice interventions thus end in impasse with patient and dentist retreating to previously held positions with respect to dental health education and the adoption of preventive actions.[2, 4, 5]

Patient-centred strategies for motivation and compliance

How can dentists enable their patients to adopt and maintain preventive health behaviours? First, it is clear that whatever strategy is to be used it must incorporate some means of providing information other than in an advice-giving format. Secondly, rather than the information being given like a prescription for some dreadful medicine, it must be presented in such a way that patients feel that it is important to them and that they can, so to speak, take ownership of it. In other words patients, within the equality of the dentist–patient relationship, can take co-ownership of the health education interaction and in doing so acknowledge their readiness to change. In such participative interactions, motivation can be perceived quite differently with patients' readiness to change acting as the key factor in promoting health skills. Readiness to change, can provide a bridge between the health care professional and patient with respect to understanding patients' lack of motivation to change their health behaviours.

Bringing about lasting and effective changes in health behaviours is not about being prescriptive but it is about participation. It is about encouraging patients to identify and express their own dental health needs, exploring their own attitudes and values as well as empowering them to make any necessary changes in their own lives. At the centre of the success of one-to-one health education is yet another partnership. This partnership is three-way. It is between the dental health professional, the patient and time. For all concerned, lasting and effective changes in health behaviours are dependent on time. The role of the health professional is to identify which patients are ready to change, and to provide them with the appropriate help and support to enable them to do so. By doing so the health professional's time can be most effectively employed, not only by enabling patients who are in a state of readiness, but also by offering other patients, who are still ambivalent, time to become ready for change. There are two procedures which are important in this regard. These are first a patient-centred technique known as motivational interviewing[2,4,5] and secondly, a framework for health actions known as the stages of change model.[6,7] Using a combination of these procedures allows dental health professionals together with their patients to accept mutual responsibility for oral health.[8] At the same time it provides the health professional with the opportunity to appreciate that change is a slow and gradual process from unawareness through motivation to compliance.

Motivational interviewing

Motivational interviewing as a patient-centred technique encourages patients to speak and by doing so enables them to identify their oral health needs. The health professional acts as a catalyst only intervening when necessary thus allowing patients to recognise resistances reflected in lifestyle barriers. It is during this initial period that the health professional starts to assess patients' ambivalence, conflict and readiness to change.

In practical terms the health professional must have a series of ground rules. These are first a fixed length of time for the appointment, secondly, to take time to explain to patients what is to happen during their times together and thirdly, to provide an environment in which patients feel able to speak, question and discuss the priority of their oral health needs. Some patients can speak freely whereas others find it difficult to start but with encouragement can overcome their reticence. However a third group exists who find it impossible to articulate their feelings. For such people the use of an 'agenda-setting chart' is essential[5] (Figure 9.1). The chart sets out a series of visual images of, for example, dental health actions for discussion. Patients choose (from the pictures) or suggest various options (as represented by the query in the blank circle) which they feel are most important to promote their oral health (Figure 9.1). In this way patients identify their own dental health goals and negotiate the time for change. Readiness to change now becomes a vital part of the process and can be assessed visually using the readiness to change ruler. This scale runs from 'not ready' through 'unsure' to 'ready'.

The motivational interviewing technique together with assessments of readiness to change, enable patients to develop their own agenda and health goals. Irrespective of whether patients feel they wish to start or not the emphasis of the motivational interview is on the individual patient. Patients' awareness of their feelings, conflicts and opinions will allow an identification of their own health goals while acknowledging their wish to change. If this is the right time for change then a personalised preventive regime may be negotiated. However when a patient is 'ambivalent' or 'not ready' then the health professional must wait. The oral health agenda and the speed of change from unawareness to compliance belongs not only with the health

Figure 9.1 To change or not to change

professional but with the patient. Therefore patients in partnership with the health professional place in motion the beginnings of their behaviour change.

Increasing awareness within a patient-centred exchange may be all that is necessary to enable a mother and child to change from unhealthy to less unhealthy behaviours. In the following example the dentist had to negotiate with the mother while acknowledging mother's fears that she had caused her daughter's dental decay. In this difficult situation the dentist had to allow the mother to state her fears. Giving advice at this point in the exchange as outlined in Case 1 would have resulted in conflict and impasse.

During the initial interview the dentist realised that Jane's mother was motivated. Mother had already thought about the reasons for her daughter's tooth decay. She had weighed up the pros and cons of removing juice as a bed-time and night-time drink and had decided that something had to be done and she was ready to change. With support from her partner at home mother was able to establish and maintain a new preventive regime for her daughter. How can dental health professionals be confident of their assessments of where their patients lie on an unawareness-compliance continuum? Such evaluations are necessary if dental health professionals are to negotiate, implement, re-negotiate and understand difficulties their patients experience when complying with preventive regimes.

Prochaska and DiClemente[6] devised a model for this eventuality. They called it the 'stages of change model'. The model is divided into six different stages of behaviour change. These are precontemplation, contemplation,

Case 1

Jane is a pretty three year old. Jane and her mother attended after Jane had a general anaesthetic to have her deciduous incisors extracted as a result of bottle caries. Jane was quite unaffected by the strange surroundings and lay quietly on mother's lap to have her teeth examined. Jane had a number of small carious lesions and so the issue of prevention needed to be addressed, in particular Jane's diet. Gently the dentist asked about it. Mother admitted that Jane was a poor eater and they had gotten into the habit of putting her to bed with 'juice'. Mother feared she was to blame, 'The juice could not have caused this it is pure — no sugar — Jane cries if she doesn't have her juice ... it's difficult to get her down at night.' Mother wanted to know how she could prevent Jane having further problems with her teeth — she was ready to change. However a conflict situation still existed which needed to be addressed. Although Mother recognised the need to prevent tooth decay she feared the difficulties she would experience if 'juice' were removed as a bed-time and night-time drink.

A solution to the problem of dental caries prevention had to be devised within the wider context of home life — that is an achievable rather than an ideal solution had to be negotiated as an interim health goal. Mother felt that Jane would tolerate a bed-time drink of milk and she would put water in the dinky cup if Jane needed a drink in the night. This solution worked with little disruption to home life. Gradually night-time drinks became unnecessary and fluoride supplement use was included in the next phase of this patient-centred preventive programme.

preparation, action, maintenance and relapse. The stages reflect and hence provide a means of assessing progress from unawareness (precontemplation) through motivation (contemplation, preparation) to compliance (action, maintenance). The stages are based upon measures of readiness to change which include the degree of ambivalence, the resolution of conflict, as well as the establishment and maintenance of the health behaviours. Thus progress through the stages is slow and torturous with many false starts and relapses. People with chronic dental problems cannot jump from precontemplation to maintenance nor can they progress in an orderly fashion from one stage to the next. Their behaviour change is characterised by forward and backward movements with progress from precontemplation to maintenance being a spiral rather than a simple linear advance.[6,7,9,10]

The stages of change model

The stages of change model can assist dental health professionals in their work with patients. It provides a framework by which they may evaluate their patients' progress from unawareness through motivation to compliance. This section describes each of the stages in detail. Clinical illustrations from practice are presented. These clinical examples demonstrate the usefulness of this technique in motivating patients to establish and maintain new health behaviours.

Stage 1: Precontemplation.

Precontemplation is characterised by patients being made aware of the need to change their health behaviours. It is at this stage that motivational interviewing as a technique is used to assess ambivalence and readiness to change. The need to acknowledge patients' ambivalence, concerns, anxieties together with their wish to change provides the dental health professional with the opportunity to set out the pros and cons of changing.[9,10] The discussion of the pros (dental health education) together with the identification of the cons (barriers) provides the basis of the precontemplation stage. Interventions used at this time must include providing patients with health information as well as the dental health professional discovering lifestyle difficulties which might act as barriers and resistances to progression to the next stage. Changes in personal health status, at this early time can act as a catalyst for progress. This was so, in the case of Mr I (Case 2) who had recently been diagnosed with maturity onset diabetes mellitus.

In this example Mr I's impetus for changing from precontemplation to contemplation was his overall physical health. Using motivational interviewing the pros and cons of changing were discussed, not only in relation to his dental health status but also in relation to his overall health. Gradually Mr I was able to move into the next stage of change.

Stage 2: Contemplation

In this stage the patient is thinking about the pros and cons of changing. The pros and cons usually have equal importance and this is illustrated in the example of Mr I. Once provided with the necessary information and his preventive strategy Mr I had to decide, to think and to contemplate what to do next. However difficulties are often encountered during this stage.[11,12] Many patients become stuck and while the pros of changing may outweigh the cons, moves to the next stage of preparation simply do not happen. These individuals have been described as 'chronic contemplators'.[11,12] Such patients are regularly seen in practice. Often children in particular can be described as chronic contemplators because although the cons of eating cariogenic snacks outweigh the pros, they are unable to give up the pleasure of carbonated drinks, confectionery, cakes and biscuits. However the example given here is of Mr C a 35-year-old married man (Case 3). He seemed

Case 2

Mr I is a 75-year-old widower. At a routine appointment the dentist noted that he had secondary caries affecting a number of his restorations. Mr I was referred to the dental hygienist for dental health education.

Discussions as to why these lesions had developed took place. Since the death of his wife Mr I had never really 'got into the way of cooking'. He got hot meals from meals-on-wheels and survived the rest of the time on sweet cups of tea with cakes and biscuits. He told the hygienist that he had been diagnosed as being diabetic but it was being controlled by diet. The hygienist using this information linked Mr I's carious teeth to his sugary snacking pattern and related it to his overall health. A preventive plan was negotiated in which the sugar was to be replaced by an artificial sweetener and the biscuits or cakes by an easily made sandwich. The hygienist continued to see Mr I. As part of his continuing care she encouraged Mr I to consult the dietician at his doctor's practice.

unable to brush his teeth effectively even after many years of oral hygiene instruction.

Stage 3: Preparation

Although many clinicians would have given up with Mr C, it seemed that the hygienist, recognised the need for a preparation time prior to Mr C being able to move into action. She felt that he needed constantly to hear the pros and cons of changing as well as participating in oral hygiene activities.[8] Cases of chronic contemplators seem to be helped by repeatedly hearing the pros and cons of changing. They are supported, encouraged and prepared for action by participating in their preventive programmes. For Mr C this meant being video-recorded while brushing his teeth. Preparation time improves self-awareness and self-image, increases readiness to change and helps in reducing the patient's ambivalence and conflict.[9–12] The need for a prolonged preparation stage seems to be essential for chronic contemplators. However their apparent lack of motivation and compliance may lead to disillusionment on the part of the dental health professional.

Stage 4: Action

By the time patients have reached the action stage they have resolved their conflict. It is as if a 'cross-over' has occurred and the pros of changing now outweigh the cons. There is the need to support the patient through these early days since the newly acquired behaviour will be subject to every possi-

Case 3

Mr C is an example of a chronic contemplator. His gingival condition was poor and his plaque scores high. Although he had attended the hygienist on many occasions and felt somewhere in himself that it was important to brush his teeth he seemed unable to put this thought into action. Nevertheless the hygienist continued to provide support and encouragement. She video-recorded Mr C while tooth-brushing believing if she gave him an active role in his prevention, he would gradually understand what he was being asked to do. He would change as she had seen others do before.

ble influence — both positive and negative (Case 4).[13]

Jim's problem in complying with his preventive regime was related to his wish to 'fit in' with his peers. It was necessary to find a solution — a compromise — and this meant retreating to the contemplation stage. The compromise solution allowed Jim to 'fit in' without his actions being entirely detrimental to his dental health status. This example illustrates the need to re-negotiate health goals as well as focusing prevention upon Jim's psychosocial needs. In this way, although the compromise health goal may not be ideal, it will be attainable and appropriate for the individual at that point in time. After all, 'health goals [are] staging posts on the way to the final destination of positive health behaviours'.[14]

Stage 5: Maintenance

Using the strategy as suggested in Case 4 enabled Jim to maintain his behaviour change. Although Jim was on the verge of relapse, using the stages of change provided all concerned with the opportunity to re-group and re-negotiate Jim's preventive programme. It is important that the intervention reflects the stage of change the patient has reached. Patients who have reached the action and maintenance stages benefit from shorter, more intensive and more participative interventions. They have taken responsibility for their oral health while acknowledging the supportive role of the dental health professional. Once action and maintenance have been reached the interventions must be 'mutually-participative' reflecting the joint responsibility for maintaining oral health improvements (Case 5).[8]

Stage 6: Relapse

Relapse occurs when maintenance strategies break down and previous unhealthy behaviours are resumed. Although this stage is common and may

Case 4

Jim is 15 years old. He is quite frightened of dental treatment and this anxiety has provided the impetus for Jim to restrict sugar to mealtimes. His mother has provided the main support for his actions. However, recently he has found it difficult to comply with his preventive programme. He plays football for the school team and after training or a match was thirsty and hungry. He feels constrained by his team-mates and so usually joins them for a fizzy drink and sugary snack. It seemed there was no way out of this difficult situation and so it was decided to retreat to the contemplation stage. The pros and cons of using sugar-free drinks and less cariogenic snacks was discussed. It was decided that he would try this option when he was next faced with peer group pressure. This interim solution has worked. All involved recognise its limitations.

appear as a disaster it provides an opportunity for re-grouping and re-negotiation of health goals. It appears that patients in the relapse phase may return to the contemplation stage but progress quickly through preparation to action.[14] Relapse allows patients to recognise that what they have achieved once, they will achieve again. The need for the health professional to be supportive and re-negotiate more realistic, achievable goals allows the patient's doubts to be expressed and conflict-changing to be resolved. According to Jacob and Plamping:[14]

> The challenge ... at the relapse stage is to be supportive and
> accepting ... to aid the patient ... re-enter the action stage rather
> than blaming her ... this has the effect of returning the patient to
> the precontemplation or contemplation stages, where she may
> question if she really wants to change anyway!

The example of Kate (Case 6) illustrates Jacob's and Plamping's concerns. Kate feared criticism and as her ambivalence increased, her readiness to change decreased. Hence there is the need to use alternative strategies. In this case a health-related approach proved fruitful. Appealing to the importance of Kate's appearance reduced Kate anger and ambivalence. This allowed Kate to appreciate the importance of changing her health behaviour.

Conclusions
There is the idea that it is easy for patients to change their health behaviours.

Case 5

Mrs F had recently had her last child. She was in her early 40s and this had been a second pregnancy within three years. She was shocked to learn that she had experienced considerable bone loss during the intervening three years. Her oral hygiene was good and she was at a loss to know how this could have happened. Discussions concerning the need for periodontal treatment on the one hand and need to maintain a rigorous level of personal oral hygiene on the other provided the opportunity to re-negotiate health goals based upon mutual participation. At this point in the intervention there was a retreat to contemplation and to preparation stages. During the preparation stage Mrs F was shown how to improve her oral hygiene using dental tape and an inter-dental brush. Periodontal care was provided. She was given support during this period in order to allow these new oral hygiene routines to become established.

All that needs to be done is to give health information and patients will change. However this disregards the inertia of mental life and the difficulties people have in changing. Many people feel ambivalent about the idea of changing since it means having to give up things which provide them with pleasure and enjoyment. If the conflict patients experience in trying to change is to be resolved then dental health professionals need to use patient-centred interviewing techniques to help them. Using motivational interviewing allows patients to explore their attitudes to both the cons (costs) and the pros (benefits) of changing as well as allowing the dental health professional the opportunity to assess their readiness to change. The patients' position on the unawareness-compliance continuum can then be assessed using the stages of change model.[6,7,9–12] This dynamic framework provides a reassurance for the health professional since it demonstrates that people can progress as well as regress through the stages.

Motivating patients to change their health behaviour is a complex issue which relies upon the understanding and patience of health professionals. By using motivational interviewing together with the stages of change model, dental health professionals can facilitate behaviour change in their patients, as well as enabling them to achieve the long-term health goals of compliance with maintenance of their newly, secured health actions.

References

1 Rosenstock I M. What research in motivation suggests for public health *Am J Pub Hlth* 1960; **50**: 295-301.
2 Rollnick S, Kinnersley P, Stott N. Methods of helping patients with behaviour change. *Br Med J* 1993; **307**: 188-190.

Case 6

Kate is an attractive 16 year old. Recently there has been an upsurge of caries activity. She has areas of decalcification between her upper incisors. Bite-wing radiographs show interstitial lesions on the premolar and molar teeth. It was clear that something has changed in Kate's diet. She was unaware that she was snacking more than usual and was angry at the implication. She had been sticking to the negotiated plan. The hygienist recognised Kate's fears that she was being blamed and so took an alternative approach — she discussed with Kate her concerns about the need for anterior restorations. Kate had an attractive smile 'it would seem a shame if she needed to have fillings in her front teeth'. Using this health-related approach enabled Kate to discuss her diet. It occurred to Kate that she had been sucking mints while studying for examinations — 'it cuts the boredom and helps me concentrate'. The effects of the mints upon Kate's teeth were discussed together with a series of sugar-free alternatives including sugar-free chewing gum. It was agreed that Kate would return to using a fluoride supplement at night. Kate was seen several times during the summer period following her examinations. The sweet eating had stopped. The hygienist's concerns about how easily Kate had relapsed were discussed with the dentist. It was decided that there was a need for continuous monitoring of Kate's compliance as an integral aspect of her oral health care.

3 Baric L. Social expectations versus personal preferences - two ways of influencing health behaviour. *J Inst Health Educ* 1977; **15**: 23-27.
4 Butler C, Rollnick S, Stott N. The practitioner, the patient and resistance to change: recent ideas on compliance. *Can Med Assoc J* 1996; **154**: 1357-1362.
5 Stott N, Rollnick S, Rees M, Pill R. Innovation in clinical method: diabetes care and negotiating skills. *Family Practice* 1995; **12**: 413-418.
6 Prochaska J O, Diclemente C C. Stages and processes of self change of smoking: toward an intergrative model of change. *Journal of Consulting and Clinical Psychology* 1983; **5**: 390-395.
7 DiClemente C C, Prochaska J O, Fairhurst S K, *et al.* The process of smoking cessation: an analysis of precontemplation, contemplation and preparation stages of change. *Journal of Consulting and Clinical Psychology* 1991; **59**: 295-304.
8 Blinkhorn A S. Factors affecting the compliance of patients with preventive dental regimes. *Int Dent J* 1993; **43**: 294-298.
9 Prochaska J O. Assessing how people change. *Cancer* 1991; **Supplement 1**: 805-807.
10 Prochaska J O. Why do we behave the way we do? *Can J Cardiol* 1995; **11 Supplement A**: 20A-25A.
11 Prochaska J O, Velicer W F, Rossi J S, *et al.* Stages of change and decisional balance for 12 problem behaviours. *Health Psychology* 1994; **13**: 39-46.
12 Velicer W F, Hughes S L, Fava J L, *et al.* An empirical typology of subjects within stage of change. *Addictive Behaviours* 1995; **20**: 299-320.
13 Brownwell K D, Cohen L R. Adherence to dietary regimens 2: components of effective interventions. *Behavioural Medicine* 1995; **20**: 155-164.
14 Jacob M C, Plamping D. *The practice of primary dental care.* London: Wright, 1989.